Why and How Doctors Kill More People than Cancer

Vernon Coleman

First Published by the European Medical Journal in 2011 as 'Do Doctors and Nurses Kill More People than Cancer?'

This book is copyright. Enquiries should be addressed to the author c/o of the publishers. This edition published on Amazon.

Copyright Vernon Coleman 2011

The right of Vernon Coleman to be identified as the author of this work has been asserted in accordance with the Copyright, Designs and Patents Act 1988.

A catalogue record for this book is available from the British Library.

For a full list of books by Vernon Coleman please see www.vernoncoleman.com or Amazon Author Central.

Contents

Boring Bit For Lawyers

Note

Dedication

Foreword

Preface: Undeniable Truths

1. A Salutary Tale Part 1: My Mother's Death

2. A Salutary Tale Part 2: My Father's Death

3. Iatrogenesis: The New Epidemic

4. The Triangle Of Evil

5. State Run Medicine Doesn't Work (The NHS Was A Terribly Stupid Idea)

6. How Hospital Staff Have Betrayed Patients

7. Doctors Are More Ignorant Than You (Or They) Think They Are.

8. Cowgirl Nurses With Great Expectations

9. Medicine Is Not A Science

10. Most Research Is Useless

11. Original Thinking Is Suppressed By The Medical Establishment

12. Most Doctors Are Addicted To Prescribing

13. The Unfair Sex

14. Killed By Prescription

15. If You Want Holistic Medicine You Must Do It Yourself

16. The NHS Has Too Much Money (But Wastes Most Of It)

17. When Trials Are Tribulations

18. If You Are Over 50 Your Government Wants You Dead

19. Your Doctor Will Kill You Now: The Cruel Waiting Game

20. Doctors Get Their Timing Wrong

21. The NHS Is Not Free

22. Bugs, Bugs, Glorious Bugs

23. The Cancer Industry: Misdirected And Ineffective

24. Travelling For Treatment

25. Cockroaches With Computers

26. Profits In Poor Countries

27. Who Lives, Who Dies?

28. Planning For Failure

29. How Sensible Living Is Penalised

30. Needless Cuts

31. Doctors Bought: Lock, Stock And Syringe Barrel

32. How And Why Doctors Ignore The Major Cause Of Illness

33. Benzo Bonanza

34. When A Vegetarian Sausage Beats An MRI Scanner

35. Committees And Quangos

36. Medical Screening Is Expensive And Doesn't Work

37. Will No One Rid Me Of The Lawyers?

38. Medical Journalists: Bought And Paid For

39. Big Brother's Evil Plan: Britain's NHS Computer Database

40. Complaints Not Wanted

41. The General Medical Council Is Worse Than Useless

42. How Lobbyists Buy Lives

43. When Simple Solutions Are Ignored

44. How The European Union Kills People

45. Looking To The Future

Postscript 1: Coleman's Laws

Postscript 2: An Interview with Vernon Coleman

Postscript 3: The Author

Boring Bit For Lawyers

These days, most books include disclaimers in which the authors apologetically warn readers that they should not rely on any information their books contain, and nor should they follow any of the advice they may find within. Disclaimers invariably go on to insist that readers who rely on anything in the book they are reading do so at their own risk. These warnings are included because the world is now full of lawyers and litigants who, under the often misguided impression that there might be money to be made, will leap at every opportunity to gouge lolly out of anyone who can be blamed for fate's little tricks. And so, as author and publisher, I warn readers that if they act on any of the facts in this book, or decide to follow any of the advice, they do so entirely at their own risk. The book has been written honestly and in good faith but I advise readers to treat facts with disdain. I recommend that advice and opinions should be disregarded or treated with great suspicion. Any reader who believes the facts in this book, or follows advice the book contains, does so entirely at their own risk. Moreover, I would also like to make it clear that books (and e-book readers) can be dangerous objects and should not be dropped, thrown or otherwise projected into areas where people or delicate objects might be damaged. In other words, dear reader, drop your e-book reader onto your toes and you're on your own.

Note

There is a tendency these days for authors to half fill their books with a list of all their sources. It is a quick and easy way to double the length of a book without doing twice as much work. It is by no means uncommon to find a book that has almost as much space devoted to lists of `references', `sources' and `notes' as is devoted to the text itself. I rather doubt if anyone (other than another author) actually bothers to consult any of these lists, which are there more to boost the author's vanity than for any other reason. The list of references is there to show the reader just how serious the author is, and how clever he or she has been. If readers don't trust the author to have done his research work properly (and to have made the appropriate deductions and drawn relevant conclusions) a list of references won't (or shouldn't) help much. When I wrote my first book (*The Medicine Men*) in 1975 my publisher, Maurice Temple-Smith, asked me whether or not I wanted to include references. He suggested that I should make a decision and stick to it for my writing career. I decided then not to waste space and money with lists of references no one would ever use. I decided that I would try to earn my readers' trust by providing them with honest, reliable reporting and with well-founded conclusions. That is what I have continued to try to do.

The truth is that scientific papers per se are often of very little value - and so references too are of dubious importance. Judgement is far more important, and it is what the reader needs. I can find scientific papers to prove virtually anything. Scientific references can be bought (some journals consist entirely of paid for articles which are of no more value than advertisements). Governments lie, drug companies lie and the medical establishment (largely bought by the first two) also lies. Interpreting what you find (and being able to read between the lines) is the key.

`In this age, the mere example of non-conformity, the mere refusal to bend the knee to custom, is itself a service. Precisely because the tyranny of opinion is such as to make eccentricity a reproach, it is desirable, in order to break through that tyranny, that people should be eccentric. Eccentricity has always abounded when and where strength of character has abounded; and the amount of eccentricity in a society has generally been proportional to the amount of genius, mental vigour, and moral courage which it contained. That so few now dare to be eccentric marks the chief danger of the time.' John Stuart Mill*

Dedication

To my Antoinette, both my rock and my haven, who shares my bewilderment, alarm and confusion in an alien world. We will always build our strength upon our steadfast love.

If God were kind and said to me

Go dream a wife

Your choice is free

She is the one who it would be.

Foreword

Things change, ideas are accepted, when the time is right. All any of us can do is to try to bring forward a little the moment when the time is right. And, in order to do that, all we can do is spread the truth and share it with everyone we know. That's why I wrote this book. I believe everything in this book is true. You may detect feelings of frustration and outrage. Those are mine but please feel free to share them. This book is published in memory of my parents who trusted much but were betrayed more. They deserved better.

Preface: Undeniable Truths

This book began as the story of my mother and father. The significance of their deaths is that most people would have thought they were normal and would have readily believed that the doctors looking after them had provided the very best of medical treatment. Most people don't know how bad health care now is. Only when you are medically trained do you really see. And most doctors (even those who understand the significance of iatrogenesis) are too cautious to criticise their own profession publicly - employed by the State they are (together with the State and the pharmaceutical industry) now part of the triangle of evil; an unholy and deadly trinity.

Nothing can bring back my parents. They are both dead. Whatever I do they are going to stay dead. And this book isn't about revenge. If I had wanted revenge I would have simply sued everyone in sight. I'm pretty sure I would have won. I wrote this book because I firmly believe that what happened to my parents happens to thousands of other patients every week. The bereaved don't know that their relatives' deaths were unnecessary because they don't know enough about medicine. They may, indeed, be grateful to the doctors and nurses for making every effort. But the fact is the case histories in this book are not exceptional. There but for the grace of God goes any one of us. And how would you, or your family know? I'm a doctor. I'm a specialist in iatrogenesis (doctor-induced disease). And yet I believe that my mother died through medical incompetence. Sadly, no one has learnt, no one has apologised and no one thinks they did anything wrong.

I wrote this book to draw attention to the fact that, for a variety of reasons, some complex and some simple, modern, State-run health care is beyond repair and now kills more people than it saves. Someone should put it out of our misery and put it to sleep. Permanently.

Today, health care is changing at a phenomenal rate. In Europe, Governments are closing small hospitals and casualty departments and concentrating services in bigger and bigger hospitals. (This is being done to please the EU whose bureaucrats believe that big is beautiful and bigger is even more beautiful). Patients who need a GP are being told to telephone for advice rather than to visit the surgery. (The excuse for this is that it will save the planet by reducing the use of petrol). Patients who are injured in accidents are told to telephone ahead and get permission in advance if they think they need to be seen in a casualty department. This may all sound bizarre. But it's true.

We need to do something.

But first we need to understand why things are so wrong with the system we have.

Today, medicine is all about making money and the people who work in State-run health care are more driven by the urge to make as much of it as possible than the people working in the so-called private sector. Doctors, nurses and administrators are in business to make as much moolah as they possibly can and don't give a toss about the patients they are supposed to care for. In July 2011, an official UK report announced that NHS managers were deliberately delaying operations in the hope that patients would remove themselves from the waiting lists `either by dying or by paying for their own treatment'. The report from the Cooperation and Competition Panel said that this tactic was one of a number used by NHS managers. At the same time GPs were being told that they were restricted in the number of referrals they could make. After threatening to collapse for years, the NHS was at last crumbling apart; aided and abetted, it has to be said, by avaricious staff members as much as incompetence. Politicians constantly boast that they are increasing the NHS budget yet again but before the Treasury has released the extra loot NHS staff will have worked out ways to divide up the spoils among themselves. Services for patients will be cut to the bone (yet again) as salaries, expenses and fees all rocket. And so the NHS becomes ever more expensive, ever more inefficient and ever more deadly.

The big issues are ignored and suppressed and those who raise them are dismissed as lunatics, heretics or fanatics. Anyone who dares to spread the truth, or raise questions, will be subjected to smear campaigns. Our liberty and our freedom of speech have been strangled by cross party consensus and an obedient media. Politicians and commentators concentrate their efforts on narrow, specific questions. The big questions, the important questions, are never asked. And so, not surprisingly, no answers are forthcoming either. Our world is controlled by the views of fifth rate politicians, Z list celebrities and bought and paid for media doctors, mouthpieces for the pharmaceutical industry.

As Texan congressman and former USA Presidential Candidate Ron Paul put it: `truth is treason in the empire of lies'. And as English philosopher Bertrand Russell once said: `In all affairs, it's a healthy thing now and then to hang a question mark on the things you have long taken for granted.'

The world's best known and longest established State-run medical service, Britain's NHS, now consists of layers of administration dedicated to deceit and committed to the principle of belligerent distortion of the truth; it practises (and is the world's best exponent of) institutionalised deception. Everything in medicine is now about money. The system exists not to protect us but to protect itself. Politicians protect the NHS because they dare not destroy it. Doctors, nurses (and other NHS workers) protect it because it protects them, feeds them and makes some of them (actually, a good many of them) exceedingly rich without their having to work too hard. This is what happens in a burgeoning fascist State. The NHS is run by incompetent people who never question their competence and so do not recognise their shortcomings. Discussions about health care never touch the real problems. Big issues (such as `Should there be an NHS?') are considered politically unacceptable so everyone involved just tinkers around the edges of the problem. No one likes to admit that the NHS is dangerous to our health or that hospitals should have a health warning hanging over their doors. The NHS stumbles along: a headless, directionless monster, kept alive by summer fętes and bring-and-by sales where local do-gooders gather together to raise cash to buy scalpels, bedpans and new bed linen.

The innocent, the naive and the well-meaning fundraisers don't realise that every penny donated protects the corrupt system and keep the whole sorry mess alive. In spirit the NHS died years ago. The shambling, disorganised, corrupt organisation which survives is a marriage between State and consumer which long ago fell apart; destroyed by the trusting naivety of the one partner and the reckless, short-sighted greed of the other. Doctors and nurses have (like long stay patients) become institutionalised. They accept everything and question nothing. They have sold their souls to the State. The NHS now kills more people than it saves. No one gives a damn about patients any more. Patients are regarded by bureaucrats, doctors and nurses as at best an inconvenience and at worst a nuisance. Everyone working for the NHS seems to have forgotten why they are there. Separating consumer from cheque writing just doesn't work in an era of selfishness, rights and unlimited expectations. There is no longer any such thing as a `public service' ethos among employees.

My fear is that everything will continue to get worse. Medical students and young nurses are being taught within a system which is geared towards defending administrators and drug companies and wherein patients are regarded (if they are regarded at all) as a nuisance. Staff are not allowed to listen to anyone (such as me) offering a realistic, honest view of what is going wrong. Doctors would much rather sweep the problems under the carpet than have the problems exposed, threatening their cosy existence. Any system which cannot cope with real criticism is corrupt.

Doctors exist only for two reasons: to look after people who have acquired a disease, and to prevent healthy people from falling ill. That's it. The rest is unimportant. They need to take back their traditional responsibility - and the authority (and power) that should always accompany responsibility. But today's medical profession has been bribed by drug companies, bullied by, and overwhelmed by, bureaucrats and social workers, and forced by politicians to abandon most of their ethical principles (including, for example, the traditional principle of confidentiality). Through the weakness of their leaders, doctors have been turned into ethically impoverished mercenaries.

This book starts with a true story, about my mother. And the book continues with another true story - this time about my father's death. I believe these stories illustrate everything that is wrong with modern medicine, they show why and how patients are being failed by a flawed system and illustrate the way in which the system protects itself with ruthless efficiency

On the pages which follow I offer a comprehensive and honest analysis of modern health care; showing precisely what is wrong and why patients are routinely cheated, endangered and killed by a system they believe they pay to protect them. State-run medicine exists to serve its staff. And it serves them well. But, as far as the system is concerned, patients are a nuisance. Britain's NHS is bigger and more corrupt and more pointlessly out of date as the Red Army.

We have sophisticated diagnostic aids, monitoring systems, thousands of drugs, microscopic surgery, lasers and a thousand and one other miracles and yet we are, by and large, over cautious, hypochondriacal, drug abusing, overweight, neurotic, constipated, nervous, neurasthenic, hysterical and unhealthy. We are a tribute to and a product of our times. And, instead of making people better, doctors are now one of the top three causes of illness. The NHS isn't a National Health Service, it's a National Homicide Service. When, to the appalling roll call of doctor-induced disease, you add the steadily increasing dissatisfaction with extended waiting lists, arrogant doctors, indifference and a lack of civility or caring it is hardly surprising that millions of people are today abandoning the traditional suppliers of medical help and seeking help from alternative practitioners.

I used to believe in the NHS.   Twenty years ago I objected strongly when friends chose to seek private medical treatment rather than use the NHS. Ten years ago I was still fighting for the NHS - although concerned about the quality of the treatment being provided for patients. But my idealistic objections to previously faithful patients betraying the NHS and having a bit on the side with the private health industry have now gone. Medicine has been ruined by political correctness, positive discrimination and targets galore.

As a result of the effect of the constant tinkering, the endless increase in layers of extra bureaucracy, the political correctness and the lawyers, a huge rift has opened up between doctors and patients. Doctors regard patients as the enemy. And patients regard doctors with distrust. Doctors are concerned only with maximising their income. In order to protect themselves from lawsuits they order batteries of investigations before daring to consider making a diagnosis. In the bad old days doctors would make diagnoses based on the patients' symptoms and their own experience and instincts. Today, diagnoses are made using tests which are far more fallible than instinct and experience. Endless laws and regulations have separated doctors from patients.

Our health care system is a failure because it is distorted by regulations, targets and legislation. Anyone who does not regard the NHS a failure should ask themselves why so many people are now flying out to India and Thailand to obtain medical care which, it is widely acknowledged, will be better and safer and much, much cheaper.

Responsibilities have been replaced by rights. And, paradoxically, the result is that in modern Britain many people, particularly the elderly, are denied treatment. Powerful organisations campaigning for particular groups of patients put pressure on the controlling political party and force the Government to provide treatment for their group. But this is done at the expense of other patients. And so politically correct groups (such as those requiring infertility treatment or sex change operations) are treated while the elderly (not at all politically correct) are allowed to go blind and to die when they could be treated quite cheaply.

Today, the NHS is a monster which causes far more deaths than traffic accidents and terrorism. It's a beast we need to kill. We will be far better off without it. A well-intentioned social experiment has been smothered by bureaucracy and the monster now exists not to care for patients but to provide secure, unchallenging employment for its staff. If the money spent on the NHS were distributed to citizens to use on private health care the *quality* of care received would soar. The UK has thousands of unemployed doctors and an NHS that is awash with administrators. Madness.

The NHS is a foul, cancerous and pustulant mess. It has been dying for years and today it is sustained by and for those who work for it and whose political future depends upon it. If it were an animal even the most loving human would have had it put down years ago. The NHS is run by people who have long since lost any genuine interest in the welfare of sick people; any compassion or sensitivity they once had has long ago been replaced by limitless self-interest. Hospitals are now run by people whose sole concern is self-preservation; they are terrified that their golden goose, overpaid and underworked employment, might be taken from them. They know that if that happens they will have to go back to being the posturing nothings they have never ceased to be. Hospitals are now managed by talentless, ignorant incompetents who destroy through egregious ineptitude. The same incompetence is shared throughout the civil service, of course, but whereas within, say, the Treasury, such incompetence merely leads to fiscal disaster, within the NHS the same level of incompetence leads to the wholesale slaughtering of the innocent. The medical establishment is controlled by people who live in a world of their own; a world where incompetence, stupidity and corruption vie for supremacy.

Finally, remember this: I'm medically qualified and, if I'm an expert on anything, it is iatrogenesis - disease that is caused by doctors. I have spent nearly half a century studying this very problem. And yet, despite my very best efforts, both my parents were, I believe, killed by the system. At the end, everything doctors did for or to my father made him worse (and eventually killed him). And nothing doctors did for my mother helped her (though I believe they could and should have saved her). As the author of *How To Stop Your Doctor Killing You* it is salutary to realise that not even I could keep my parents alive. How many other people are being killed by doctors? The only certainty is that it is far, far more than the figures suggest. I firmly believe that doctors and nurses now kill more people than cancer.

Neither of my parent's deaths was recognised as `medical accidents' by the system. If I hadn't been a doctor I wouldn't have noticed anything wrong with the two deaths.

Today, drug-reliant medicine has spread as the public relations departments of large multinational drug companies have worked overtime to convince doctors and patients that drugs are the only way to prevent and treat disease. Massive drug and vaccination programmes have begun. Doctors have been bought in their thousands and now preach the drug company gospel. In the USA and the UK, and just about every other country in the world, drug companies now control doctors. It is no coincidence that iatrogenesis is now one of the top three causes of disease and death. Doctors and drugs can be useful. They can save lives. But they must be treated with caution - as though they were, like cigarettes, labelled with a Government health warning.

We all have a responsibility to take personal charge of our own health and destiny. We must become health care consumers - able to make the most important decisions ourselves and to pick and choose which treatments to accept and which to reject. We must use doctors as technicians - there to advise and provide technical support - but we must learn how and when to make the big decisions ourselves.

It is the ultimate purpose of this book (and indeed of all my medical books) to help readers become independent health care consumers. Welcome to the medical revolution.

Vernon Coleman, August 2011

1. A Salutary Tale Part 1: My Mother's Death

In October 2004 my mother had difficulty in walking. When she was first admitted to Royal Devon and Exeter hospital in Exeter, she was thought to need extensive physiotherapy to help her walk again. She was mentally alert. In November 2004, after a rapid deterioration, it was decided that my mother was suffering from terminal cancer with metastases. She was not considered healthy enough for palliative radiotherapy. She was described, by her consultant oncologist, as `frail, confused, bedbound and dependent'. She had to be catheterised because she was incontinent. The idea of rehabilitation was abandoned because of her alleged terminal cancer. A neurologist who assessed her mental state reported that my mother did not know where she was and had failed to recognise the doctor. She was given the usual simple mental test (date of birth and so on) and scored 0 out of 10. My father was telephoned at home and told that my mother was terminally ill with cancer and that there were metastatic deposits in her spine, lung and possibly liver. It was thought that her mental condition could be caused by secondaries in her brain. No one knew what sort of cancer she was suffering from or where the primary was situated. My father was telephoned and told that a breast cancer she had many years earlier, and from which she had officially recovered, had suddenly recurred, though there was absolutely no evidence for this theory. (Following an operation to remove a breast, she had refused chemotherapy and radiotherapy after asking to see evidence that the proposed treatment might be suitable for a woman of her age. Although she was over 70 at the time she was only given evidence showing that the suggested treatment might be suitable for premenopausal women. My mother, who had left school at 14, could see at a glance that this wasn't of much relevance to her. She decided that `it's what we do' didn't count as a scientific explanation and so she and my father decided that she'd pass on those, thank you very much for offering. She made a complete recovery but as she lay in her hospital bed various members of staff blamed the cancer. My father was devastated. The diagnosis caused him untold grief, soul-searching and guilt. (It turned out that the people who told him this were quite wrong. My mother's illness and her death had absolutely nothing to do with the breast cancer.)

I telephoned the cancer specialist. She told me that my mother either had cancer of the breast or the lung with secondaries and was too weak for treatment. `That's the nature of the beast', she said. She told me that there was no hope but did agree that the registrar's action in telephoning my father when he was at home alone was barbaric.

On Sunday 21st November we noticed that my mother's urine bag was red. There was clearly blood in her urine. A nurse had changed the catheter bag several times without bothering to report to anyone that the urine in the bag was red with blood. Or perhaps they hadn't noticed. I reported the blood and a doctor put my mother on amoxicillin for a urinary infection. After the blood appeared in the urine the cancer specialist told me that my mother had secondaries in her kidneys. By the 30th November the urine was clear and the bag was no longer red. The diagnosis of cancer secondaries in the kidneys was never withdrawn, though it too was wrong.

My mother stayed in the Exeter hospital, which is a teaching hospital, for the next few months. Numerous consultants saw her and decided that there was nothing to be done. Her symptoms now seemed to defy diagnosis. She managed to get out of bed occasionally but was unsteady on her feet. And she had developed a rather strange way of walking with her feet wide apart.

My wife, Antoinette, who has no medical training, put my mother's symptoms into an Internet search engine. She came up with several differential diagnoses. From the short list she produced we both agreed that normal pressure hydrocephalus was the most likely diagnosis. I'd never heard of it but the disease fitted my mother's symptoms perfectly.

She had an unusual wide-legged walk. She had a tendency to fall. And she had urinary incontinence. She was also showing signs of dementia. These are precisely the symptoms shown by patients with normal pressure hydrocephalus. *Precisely*.

Normal pressure hydrocephalus is not something GPs see very much. But it is the sort of thing teaching hospital neurologists really should know about. I had never seen a patient with it. The doctors looking after my mother listened politely to my suggestion that they consider normal pressure hydrocephalus but immediately dismissed it and stuck with their neoplastic madness. There was never a shred of evidence in support of that diagnosis.

During the period when my mother was lying in her hospital bed in Bolham Ward in Exeter I made a few notes. Here are some of them:

1. An emergency door at the end of the ward had three bolts securing it in addition to a lock and a padlock. When my father mentioned that this didn't seem a very good idea for an emergency exit the staff solved the problem by removing the notice describing the door as an emergency fire exit. The door remained bolted, locked and padlocked.

2. When a drip bottle needed changing a warning beep sounded for more than 10 minutes. Eventually I went and found a nurse to change it. I don't know what would have happened if I hadn't been there.

3. On numerous occasions my mother didn't see a doctor of any description between Friday and Monday. The hospital seemed to pretty much close down at weekends. During the week doctors never seemed to be available after 5.00 p.m.

4. I watched a nurse take a pulse with a machine. She recorded the pulse rate but didn't bother to note that my mother's pulse rate was irregular.

5. No nurse ever brushed my mother's hair or did her make up. Her hair was only ever combed when we visited. She was aware of this

and felt ashamed. When my dad told her that some visitors were coming she cried and tried to brush her hair with her fingers.

6. On at least one occasion in November 2004 the staff didn't bother to give my mother any food because they said `she was too weak to eat'.

7. A hospice nurse went to see my mother and told her: `You aren't fit enough for radium treatment/radiotherapy'. My mother didn't know that she was suspected of having cancer so this came as something of a surprise to her. She didn't understand why she'd been told this.

8. Whenever we visited my wife had to take my mother to the lavatory. We had to help her in and out of bed by ourselves.

9. The hospital's internal mail system seemed pathetic. On one occasion it took four days to move an item from the X-ray department to the ward. It would have been far quicker to use second class post.

10. My mother spent virtually all her time in bed. From Thursdays until Tuesdays she usually saw no physiotherapist and had no help in moving about. She just lay in bed becoming weaker and losing all confidence in her own body. After I complained the physiotherapists turned up for a meeting. I was told that there weren't enough physiotherapists to give her the care she needed. We couldn't move my mother to a private hospital because she has not yet been diagnosed and clearly a private hospital would not have the investigative wherewithal. When I asked if I could send in private physiotherapists I was told that I could not. It occurred to me that the nurses on the ward had not heard of the danger of deep vein thrombosis or the need to avoid pressure sores by moving patients around.

11. On one occasion the fire alarm went off at 4.00 a.m. but no one came. My mother, who was at that point still fairly coherent and alert, lay in bed absolutely petrified. Even if she had been able to get out of bed she wouldn't have been able to leave the ward very easily

because the fire exit door was padlocked. No one ever came and eventually the fire alarm went off without explanation.

12. On one occasion an elderly man lay naked on his bed with the door wide open. On occasion my mother would also throw off all her clothes and we would have to rush to draw the screens while we fought to pull the bed covers over her. The nurses didn't come because whoever had designed the ward had positioned the nurses' station in such a way that it was difficult if not impossible for them to see what was happening.

13. On several occasions I watched a cleaner take a broom for a walk down the middle of the ward. She didn't bother cleaning under the beds or around them.

14. A female patient in a bed opposite to my mother pressed the button for a nurse because she needed a bedpan. No one came and I couldn't find a nurse anywhere. Eventually the woman, full of shame, said, plaintively: `It's too late now.'

15. On one occasion I sat beside my mother's bed when two nurses arrived. One said: `Have you had a cup of tea this morning? `Yes thank you,' said my mother, who had been officially declared demented and mentally incompetent. `Right.' said the nurse. She wrote this information down on the fluids chart she was carrying. The cup of tea was standing, untouched, on the bed table in front of my mother. If we hadn't helped her drink I firmly believe that my mother would have died of dehydration.

At one point during her stay in the Exeter hospital my mother improved noticeably after she had a diagnostic lumbar puncture and some cerebrospinal fluid was removed. I thought that the improvement might be significant. It was the only time during her stay in Exeter that she showed any signs of improvement. For a day or two she seemed stronger and her mental function even began to improve a little. It seemed to me to suggest that there had been too much fluid around my mother's brain. Maybe the lumbar puncture, by removing some of the fluid, had reduced the pressure and alleviated her symptoms. Maybe the diagnosis of normal pressure hydrocephalus was correct after all. The doctors to whom I mentioned this dismissed my suggestion and insisted that the improvement was simply a coincidence. What would a former GP and writer of books know about these things? No one actually patted me on the head but it felt as though they had done so.

After my mother had finally been diagnosed as suffering from normal pressure hydrocephalus (just before she died) I checked with a large medical textbook. Here is what it says: `To help with the diagnosis, doctors do a spinal tap (lumbar puncture) to remove excess cerebrospinal fluid. If this procedure relieves symptoms, normal pressure hydrocephalus is likely, and treatment is likely to be effective.'

There are very few devastating diseases that can be cured so cheaply, so quickly and so permanently.

In the spring of 2005 my mother was still in the hospital and her condition had deteriorated. On Monday 25th April 2005 I saw the neurology registrar at the Royal Devon and Exeter hospital who confirmed that my mother's prognosis was bleak. The hospital staff still hadn't made a diagnosis. The cancer diagnosis had been forgotten. I was told that six neurologists and numerous other consultants had seen her. Every conceivable test had been done. The registrar told me that it would be difficult to find a nursing home capable of looking after her. In addition to her physical paralysis she was again diagnosed as suffering from dementia. I was told that this could be vascular or a consequence of possible encephalitis. It seemed clear that my mother needed to stay in hospital for the rest of her life.

    I was advised that there were no nursing homes in Budleigh capable of looking after my mother. Afterwards we sat by my mother's beside. Antoinette, my wife, was feeding my mother. I sat on the other side of the bed. As we left my mother pulled her urine catheter bag out from under the bedclothes and tried to blow her nose with it.

On Tuesday 26th April 2005 my mother was, at my request, moved to Budleigh hospital so that my father, who lived in Budleigh, could visit more easily. For six months he had visited the Exeter hospital once or twice a day to feed my mother (who would otherwise have almost certainly starved to death). I also wanted my mother out of the hospital in Exeter because I wasn't terribly impressed by the nursing care she had received. If I had to choose two words to describe the hospital care they would be `apathetic' and `neglectful'.

On Wednesday 27th April, at 9.00 p.m., someone from Budleigh hospital telephoned my father (who is 85) and asked him when he would be moving his wife out of the hospital. This was the second time he'd received an evening telephone call that had frightened him out of his wits. My mum had been in the hospital for just slightly more than 24 hours. No one there had made any attempt to make a diagnosis. It didn't strike me as the sort of hospital that does terribly much in the way of diagnostic work. It was, it seemed to me, what used to be called a cottage hospital.

My father was startled and shocked by the suddenness and timing of the telephone call asking him when he would be moving mother out of the hospital. He got the impression that the hospital was planning to send my mum home for him to look after by himself. She was incapable of doing anything for herself. She was doubly incontinent, required nursing on a ripple bed and had been diagnosed as demented. She had to be kept in a bed with cot sides so that she didn't fall onto the floor. On the odd occasion when she tried to feed herself she ended up with food everywhere - with the result that both she and the bed had to be changed. My mother was so incapable of moving by herself that the nurses had a hoist and a bed lift fitted to the bed so that they could move my mother around and in and out of bed. It took two nurses to move her up the bed. She needed constant nursing attention.

My wife and I were in France when my mother was moved to the hospital in Budleigh. We came straight back and visited the hospital the next day, Thursday the 28th. Within five minutes of my arriving at my mother's bedside a nurse asked me to go to the sister's office. A nurse wanted to know when my mother would be leaving the hospital. My mother had, by then, been in the hospital for no more than 48 hours. I found the questioning cruel, unfeeling and inhumane. Throughout my mother's stay I found the hospital staff aggressive and offensive.

My father, who had been in a state of shock, now became depressed as a result of the hospital's attitude. Up until Monday the 25th April, my father had hoped that he would be able to have my mother back home or that, at the very least, he would be able to take her out of the hospital for trips in a wheelchair. He had been making plans to buy a motorised chair and a suitable vehicle so that he could do this. He thought a week or two in the hospital would lead to her returning home.

When I spoke to the nurse at Budleigh Hospital on 28th April 2005 I was told that an assessment had been done and that my mother was considered fit to move out of the hospital and was now regarded as mentally alert. My mother had, according to Budleigh Hospital, been cured from her dementia within two days. She had received no new treatment. She had merely been moved to a local small town hospital. The nurse admitted that my mother needed nursing care but insisted that mentally there was nothing wrong with her. The hospital had, she told me, already applied for an enforcement order to have my mother removed from the hospital. I was shocked by their ruthlessness.

In reality, there had been no change whatsoever in my mum's condition. Several neurologists at Royal Devon and Exeter hospital had already agreed that my mother was suffering from severe dementia and though it turned out that they had missed the primary diagnosis there wasn't much doubt that a diagnosis of dementia was understandable - at least it would have been if it had been a diagnosis made by a nurse or a member of the public. Through a mixture of stubbornness and stupidity the highly paid hospital specialists had missed the crucial diagnosis (even though it had been handed to them on a plate) but neither we nor anyone at the Budleigh hospital knew that.

I complained about the fact that my father had been rung at home the evening before but the nurse didn't seem to think that there was anything wrong with that. She didn't apologise. I wanted to know just how ill you had to be to be in hospital these days. I felt overwhelmed with guilt. I had arranged for my mother to be moved to the Budleigh Hospital so that my father could visit more easily. And now they wanted to throw her out. But where could we take her? I went back to sit by mother's bed. As I sat down my mother looked up and pointed to a stranger on the other side of the ward. `Is that Vernon over there?' she enquired. We were living a nightmare. She didn't know who I was. She didn't recognise my wife. And she often wasn't sure who my father was. When I talked to her she didn't even know that she was in hospital. Somewhere in the hospital a bell rang. `There's someone at the door,' she said.

Someone at the Budleigh hospital threatened to send my mother home in an ambulance, even though they knew that my father could hardly look after himself. They also knew that my mother needed intensive nursing care. My mother was, said one snotty little bastard, terminally but not finally terminally ill. It was the first time I'd heard the phrase. My father, in his mid 80s, was devastated. `What do I do if they send her home?' he asked. `Don't answer the door,' I told him. `Don't let them into the house. Call me.' I was telling my father to refuse to let the ambulance men bring my mother into the house. It was awful, just bloody awful. If the plan was to put us under pressure it was working very well. I'd never seen my father so distraught. My mother's GP at the time, Dr Taylor, agreed that we would not be able to find a local nursing home capable of looking after her. No one at the Budleigh hospital seemed to me to give a damn what happened to my mother as long as she wasn't their responsibility.

As far as I am aware no one made the slightest attempt to make a diagnosis during the time my mother was in the Budleigh Hospital. Since they didn't want to nurse her and they didn't do any diagnostic tests it's difficult to see the point of the hospital - apart from providing employment for the staff.

On the 11th May I had to attend a meeting at Budleigh hospital to discuss my mother's expulsion from the hospital. I was told that the hospital did not have enough beds and desperately needed to get rid of my mother. There were four people at the meeting: two members of the nursing staff, someone who looked like an administrator and Dr Taylor, my mother's GP at the time. I mistakenly thought that he at least would be on my parents' side. I was disappointed. The meeting was held in a completely empty ward. There were plenty of beds, all empty, and it seemed to me that this wasn't the first time the empty ward had been used for a meeting. If the hospital was short of anything it was patients, not beds.

The meeting lasted an hour and it turned out to be one of the most unpleasant hours of my life. I have been grilled by some of the country's toughest television and radio interviewers. I have given evidence in the House of Lords and the House of Commons but nothing prepared me for this. For a solid hour the four of them battered at me to take my mother out of the hospital. They used every manipulative and emotional trick in the book. I quickly realised that no one there cared a damn about my mother or my father. They just wanted to get rid of a patient who seemed likely to be a long-term expense. This was business. I was still desperate to try to find a diagnosis. I was still trying to support my father. I was grieving for my mother who no longer even recognised me. I was told that my mother would be better off in a nursing home and that the hospital didn't have any long-stay beds. I was told that they needed the bed for other patients (no one seemed to see the irony in the fact that the meeting was being held in a completely empty ward) and that my father would be better off if my mother was elsewhere. They didn't explain how this could be when there was no nursing home for miles that would be able to cope with her needs. My father lived near to the hospital and could easily visit within minutes. I was told that my mother would be better off in a private room. I pointed out that she couldn't read or watch television or listen to the radio. She had no memory or mental capacity. I pointed out that being in a hospital ward gave her things to watch. I knew that being in a small, closed room would be awful for her. No one seemed to give a damn. I was told that my mother was more at risk of catching an infection in a hospital (the only thing I agreed with). At the end of the meeting they told me that they couldn't agree to my mother staying in the hospital and that she had to leave. I left the meeting and went back to my mother's bedside. She was still unable to move. She still didn't know who she was or where she was. She didn't know who I was. She was still faecally incontinent. She still had a catheter in her bladder to collect her urine. She still had to be fed. She still couldn't walk or even wash herself. But according to the hospital staff she was fine and mentally alert. I wondered if they wanted to throw my mother out because they knew we could afford the nursing home fees. Ageism is the new racism: no respect, no consideration, no courtesy, no dignity, no caring. The whole penny pinching exercise was made even more heartless and unforgivable by the fact that I know that hospital staff waste billions through incompetence. Billions are stolen and frittered away by the wicked statist guardians we pay to look after us.

For several weeks after that my father didn't dare visit my mother at all. He was frightened that he would again be pressured by the staff to move my mother. He didn't know where he could take her. He was overwhelmed with grief and now he was tortured by guilt and anxiety.

Another mental assessment was done on my mother. It was a sick joke. The assessor asked my mother what I did for a living. My mother thought for a while. `He's a teacher,' she said at last. She didn't know who I was, let alone what I did for a living. `That's close enough,' answered the assessor putting a tick in another box. My mother was declared mentally competent. On the 19th July my mother complained to me that two dogs had been fighting on the ward. On the 22nd July my father was sitting by my mother's side when the vicar called. My mother told him they were waiting for a train. The vicar thought it was a joke but my mother was serious. She kept asking my father why the train wasn't there. My mother didn't recognise my father or know what he'd done for a living. She didn't know anything. She didn't even know who she was or where she was. She held her head a good deal though and it was clear that she was having constant headaches. (No one at the hospital realised that these were caused by the increase in the amount of fluid surrounding her brain.)

On the 27th July I attended another meeting in Budleigh Hospital. This time there were nine people there representing the hospital and the NHS. Nine of them. Dr Graham Taylor, my mother's GP was there, together with two nurses, a 'continuity care manager', an 'acting leading continuity nurse', a 'hospital care manager', a 'discharge facilitator', a representative of the administrators and a representative from Exmouth social services. I wrote down all their names. Someone began by saying that they all had my mother's best interests at heart. Someone else said they were delighted to report that my mother was much better and was improving. I asked them why, if this was the case, they weren't giving her any occupational therapy or physiotherapy. No one had an answer to this. I got the impression they thought it was an unfair question. I asked them how they had managed to produce this miracle without any treatment. I wanted to know how a woman who had been officially declared terminally ill and demented and in need of constant care had suddenly become `physically capable and mentally alert' after a few weeks in a small town hospital. No one had any answers. In fact, of course, when the final diagnosis was made it was quite clear that my mother could not possibly have shown any physical or mental improvement. She was suffering from normal pressure hydrocephalus which was steadily getting worse. And very early on in the illness she had been officially declared to be demented.

The hospital staff who said that she had recovered and could be discharged were completely wrong. I find it difficult to avoid the suspicion that they said she was better simply because they wanted to throw my mother out of the hospital. Bizarrely, the continuity care manager wanted proof that I represented my mother and made what he called a formal objection to the fact that I had not given them my home address. When I pointed out that my mother needed intensive nursing care he claimed, to my utter astonishment, that catheters, hoists and ripple beds were not medical equipment. I asked him what would count as medical equipment. He said a ventilator would count as medical equipment. So, presumably, if my mother had been on a ventilator they wouldn't have wanted to throw her out. One of the 'nine' said that they only paid for the care of patients who were in the final stage of cancer. The phrase 'final stage terminally illness' was used. And again I heard the phrase 'terminally, terminally ill'. I asked how they knew that a patient was terminally, terminally ill and was told that they could tell this through liver and kidney deterioration. I asked if they had done any tests to check on this and it was generally agreed that they couldn't remember whether any such tests had been done. I got the impression they seemed to think the question was embarrassing and therefore unfair. I have no idea why nine people wasted a good chunk of a day on such a pointless meeting. I hate to think what it must have cost. It occurred to me as I sat there that if they were all sacked there would be plenty of money left for looking after patients and I told them that the bullying had won and that we would take my mother out of the hospital so that they could have yet another empty bed. I don't think I ever saw any of the nine again.

According to the law the NHS had a full responsibility for looking after my mother. According to the relevant legislation the NHS was expected to arrange and fund rehabilitation and recovery services and palliative care. It is inconceivable that my mother did not fulfil the eligibility criteria for continuing NHS healthcare. The law is clear: if the primary need for care is due to severe ill health, then all costs of nursing, personal care and accommodation should be funded by the State health service. Today, on reflection, it seems to me that the nine people at the meeting at Budleigh Hospital had become institutionalised and were working for the system and not for patients.

In the end my father couldn't bear it any longer. I really couldn't blame him. The staff at the Budleigh Hospital were making us feel so unwelcome, and harassing us so much, that we had no choice but to move my mother. As far as the NHS was concerned it was all about money. They wanted to avoid the cost of looking after my mother - even though they had a moral and legal responsibility to do so. My father, my wife and I all knew that moving my mother out of the hospital was the wrong thing to do for her because she needed the hospital environment but in the end my father just couldn't cope with the pressure. I don't blame him. We found the Cranford Nursing Home, a private nursing home in Exmouth, which could cope. For around Ł750 a week my mother had a private room which seemed crowded with three adults visiting. My wife and felt that the en suite `bathroom' was more like a cupboard and we both felt that if a hotel had offered us the room we would have walked out in disgust.

My father sold his home and bought a small house near to the nursing home so that he could visit regularly. My mother was tearful when she moved into the nursing home. She had hardly spoken for months. But she spoke now. The first thing she said was: `I don't like it here.' Because much of their money was in joint accounts, and my mother couldn't sign her name, my father had to arrange for a power of attorney so that he could access their savings and pay the nursing home fees. (Even this was not always accepted, and my dad had no choice but to forge my mum's signature.)

My mother died in the nursing home. The diagnosis had by then been made. Numerous consultants (including several neurologists), countless junior hospital doctors, one or two GPs and a good many nurses all missed the diagnosis. (Since nurses now want to be regarded as almost equal to doctors they must take some of the blame). We watched my mother die a terrible, slow death. She died because the doctors failed to make the diagnosis until it was too late.

Towards the end of her life we visited my mother in the nursing home and as soon as Antoinette entered the room she turned to me and said that my mother had a swollen, bulging eye. The diagnosis now was beyond doubt. My mother had a bulging eye because of the pressure inside her skull. I contacted my mother's new GP and asked him to arrange for my mum to go back into Exeter hospital. I don't think he or any of the people looking after my mother in the nursing home had realised the significance of this. In the Royal Devon and Exeter Hospital the doctors at last confirmed the diagnosis of normal pressure hydrocephalus. It was the diagnosis we'd offered them within a month of my mother falling ill. It had taken endless NHS doctors and two NHS hospitals to reach the diagnosis. If they'd acted within days or even weeks of her being admitted then they could have saved her life. Treatment for normal pressure hydrocephalus is easy, fast, cheap and effective. A shunt is placed in the ventricles of the brain and run under the skin. Cerebrospinal fluid is then drained away from the brain. This procedure will then significantly improve the symptoms.

But by now it was too late. On the death certificate my mother's death is recorded as dementia with normal pressure hydrocephalus as the underlying problem. I never told my dad how my mother could have been saved. It was, for my mother, a slow and painful and humiliating death. If it can happen to my family it can happen to yours. Remember, it is only because I am a doctor (and my wife is an excellent researcher) that we finally managed to persuade the doctors to (belatedly) reach the correct diagnosis. Remember that in order to save money NHS staff in Budleigh insisted that my mother was rational and mentally alert (when she was suffering from dementia). Remember, too that we failed to save my mother's life. She was killed by incompetence. No one has ever apologised. No one has ever admitted that any mistakes were made. And I have no doubt that no one ever will.

These days I am always nervous about spending time in the Exeter region in case either my wife or I fall ill. After all, as you will see, I believe that the medical services in South Devon successfully 'killed' both my parents. The hospital where my parents were treated so appallingly is a teaching hospital for young doctors. And there is some irony in the fact that one employee of the local medical school has been a violent critic of alternative medicine. Heaven knows what they teach at the Royal Devon and Exeter hospital. I sincerely hope it has nothing to do with medicine. I haven't been to enough hospitals to be able to say that it's the worst in the world but if there is one worse I sincerely hope, for the sake of future patients, that the staff are soon carried off by aliens.

2. A Salutary Tale Part 2: My Father's Death

My father was an inventor, company director and World War II naval veteran. He died on February 28th 2008. He was 87-years-old. The inquest into his death was held in Exeter. Although the inquest was held at my request I did not attend. This is the extraordinary, astonishing, almost unbelievable story of his death and of what followed.

At around 4.00 a.m. on the morning of 5th February 2008 my father got up out of bed and made himself a drink. The pain in his back was terrible and he was having trouble breathing. It wasn't a new pain. He'd had it before. This time the pain seemed to be mainly referred to his lower ribs at the front of his chest. Knowing that if he rang too soon he would get the emergency medical service and probably be told to take two aspirin and ring his doctor in the morning, he waited until around 9.00 a.m. to telephone his doctor. (The fact that he waited five hours before calling a doctor suggested to me that the pain couldn't have been too bad and that, maybe, a home visit might have been more appropriate.) He told me that he had a bad night because he had got himself into an uncomfortable position. He needed to see the doctor but didn't feel up to driving to the surgery. He had a long-standing problem with his back: as the GP should have known, he had chronic osteoporotic spine pain which caused pains all around his chest.

My father telephoned Dr Benjamin Hallmark at Budleigh Salterton Medical Centre. My father was, according to Dr Hallmark, complaining of excruciating pain. But instead of visiting, Dr Hallmark simply told my father (in excruciating pain, remember) to dial 999 and arrange for himself to be taken to hospital in an ambulance. The doctor didn't even bother to make the telephone call.

I believe that if Dr Hallmark had visited, my father might still be alive today - largely because he almost certainly would have decided that my dad did not require hospitalisation. I'm old-fashioned and still believe that a GP has a duty to visit patients who call for help. (Even if an ambulance is also considered necessary.) And my father might still be alive today because it was the sequence of events which followed which led, I believe, to his death. It was, in retrospect, the first of many unfortunate decisions. And it was the beginning of a sequence of disastrous events which would lead to his death just over three weeks later.

My father was taken to Royal Devon and Exeter Hospital where he was given extensive tests. The doctors looking after him confirmed that there was no heart problem. No serious or new problems were found. This wasn't very surprising. At no point had my father ever had any symptoms of a heart attack. My father still had some pain and asked if he could have more morphine. The ambulance crew had given him some and he had, he said, rather liked the feeling. The doctors with him (a consultant and a junior hospital doctor) instantly said that he didn't need morphine. They told him that paracetamol or codeine would control his pain. The consultant said that he could go home the following day. My father seemed quite well. He was very alert. At one point I remember him asking the consultant to fetch him a telephone directory. The admitting consultant considered sending my father home again. He decided, however, to keep him in overnight. I know all this because as soon as I heard what had happened I drove to Exeter and I was standing by my father's bedside at the time. My father was quite well, sitting up in bed taking a very active interest in what was happening. He was most concerned that I should get in touch with a friend with whom he had a luncheon appointment.

The following day my dad asked the doctors if they could do anything about his breathing problems. More investigations were ordered. He was expected to be in hospital no more than another day or possibly two. And then the ward was infected with a diarrhoea and vomiting bug and was closed. My father was effectively imprisoned in the hospital. Because the ward was closed there were no physiotherapists, no occupational therapists and no visitors. I tried to get him moved to a nearby private hospital. But they wouldn't take him because he was on an infected ward. The nursing home wouldn't take him for the same reason.

In the next ten days or so he was (I believe) twice infected with a diarrhoea and vomiting bug. He also contracted a chest infection and a urinary tract infection. (The latter developed after he was catheterised. He was catheterised because, like most 87-year-old men, he had been getting up at night to pass urine. Unfortunately, he got an infection and they had to take the catheter out. In my view, anyone who gets a urinary infection from a simple catheterisation has been catheterised by a nincompoop.) The staff insisted that the diarrhoea and vomiting bug was airborne (so it wasn't their poor hygiene which caused the persistent spread). I didn't believe them then and I don't believe them now. Such bugs are largely spread through poor hygiene practices. If the staff really believed the bug was airborne why weren't they wearing masks? And why were the doors to the ward left wide open? A doctor said the bug was spread by projectile vomiting and this can be true. But that doesn't make it an airborne infection - unless, of course, one patient vomits directly into the mouth of another. It didn't seem surprising to me that they were having difficulty controlling the infection. One `expert' told me that such bugs behave differently in hospitals though they couldn't explain how the bugs know they are in a hospital. The real problem is: if you don't know how an infection is transmitted how do you stop it? (The staff suffer from these bugs less than the patients because they don't eat on the ward and don't use the same lavatories.)

I wasn't impressed by the quality of care provided. I was told by one member of staff that my dad had diarrhoea because of the codeine he was taking. (Codeine is more likely to cause constipation). I heard a doctor ask another patient how his bowels were. When told that they were runny the doctor said she would prescribe a laxative.

Although the ward was closed I visited my dad on 15th February. I was allowed to visit because he had suddenly become very ill. When I visited him I found that he was very pink, confused and twitching. When he did wake up he had difficulty in seeing. He was on oxygen and it seemed pretty clear to me that he was getting too much of the stuff and was suffering from oxygen poisoning. These are all classic symptoms of this problem. I asked for the oxygen to be stopped. The oxygen was stopped and the following morning my father was fine.

I spent much of the following week struggling to get my dad out of the hospital. I spoke to him and the staff several times a day, every day. His pain was controlled and he was bored and fed up. I spoke countless times to doctors and nurses on the ward. Eventually, after a flurry of calls on Friday 22nd February, I managed to arrange for my dad (who no longer had the virus and was now safely in a side room) to be moved to the Cranford Nursing Home near to his home to convalesce. He was told that the additional tests they had not been able to do (because of the ward closure) would be conducted as an outpatient. By this time my father wasn't fit enough to go to his own home. He needed physiotherapy to help him walk again. After two weeks in hospital he had become very weak, though he was still mobile. His spare pyjamas went with him to the nursing home, in a bag. When the bag was opened the pyjamas were thickly stained with the diarrhoea he had suffered on the ward. Not the best way to stop infections spreading.

The hospital had prescribed a regime to control my father's pain and given him an outpatient appointment for further investigations of his long-term respiratory problem. I was told that after admission to the nursing home he was laughing and joking with the nurses.

I had influenza and was too ill to visit him that weekend (I didn't want to give him the infection I'd acquired) but I spoke to him several times and he seemed well enough. I thought he was safe now that he was out of the hospital. He received visitors and had his television set moved across from his house. He walked about in the nursing home (he walked so much he made himself tired - he told me that he thought he had overdone things) and I asked him if he thought he would still be able to come away with us for a few days in Sidmouth to celebrate his birthday (3rd March). He said he would and that he was looking forward to it.

My dad wasn't ready to die. He was looking forward to all sorts of things. We'd just brought him a new printer and fax machine for his birthday and a new gadget-packed mobile phone. Before going into hospital he still drove himself and went out to lunch several times a week.

When he was discharged from the hospital my father's pain was controlled with a Fentanyl patch. He was, I believe, on a relatively low dose of this. Much stronger patches could have been tried. But on 25th February the nursing home staff called his doctor, Dr Hallmark, because he was again complaining of pain.

The doctor who called on Dr Hallmark's behalf, was a GP registrar, Dr Stuart Livingston. He overruled the regime which had been carefully prepared by the hospital doctors who had looked after my dad for two weeks and prescribed Oramorph (morphine). The manufacturers of Oramorph state clearly that the drug should not be given to patients with severe respiratory problems. It's a serious hazard. The drug is a version of morphine and it depresses respiration. Michael Jackson is said to have died of an opiate induced respiratory arrest. And my dad was 87-years-old. In old age drug effects can be dramatically enhanced. Two days later - after several doses of Oramorph - my father was dead. Dr Livingston stated in his report to the coroner, Dr Elizabeth Earland, in support of his action, that he believed the contraindication to be a relative rather than an absolute one. The manufacturer of the drug, however, makes it clear that the contradiction is absolute. To be precise, the company making Oramorph told me: `...the use of Oramorph is contraindicated in any patients with respiratory depression or obstructive airways disease regardless of age.' My father had chronic obstructive pulmonary disease - a serious respiratory problem. Dr Livingston also suggested that prescribing Oramorph is acceptable in `end stage' respiratory disease. But my father was not `end stage' anything. I don't believe that Dr Livingston had ever met my father before he prescribed Oramorph for him. My father didn't even think of himself as old. A few weeks earlier he had gone to a club for pensioners and had complained bitterly about it. `It's full of old people,' he muttered sourly. He had been driving his car the day before he was admitted to hospital.

When I telephoned him at 9.00 a.m. on Wednesday morning (27th February) my dad was very sleepy and kept falling asleep during our conversation. I put the telephone down and rang a little later. He was still very drowsy, seemed drugged, and had difficulty in breathing. I had spoken to him virtually every day for four years and I had never heard him have as much trouble with his breathing as he had after that day. I guessed that his medication had been changed and asked him what new drug he was on. He told me that he had seen a GP on Monday who had given him morphine. I spoke immediately to a senior member of staff and asked him not to give my father any more of the morphine. I was told that the morphine had been prescribed four times a day and as required. I was horrified and pointed out that since morphine is a respiratory depressant and my father was suffering from severe respiratory problems the morphine would kill him. The staff member agreed that no more morphine would be given. I said I would take responsibility for stopping the morphine and he accepted this. I said I would visit the following day (Thursday).

I telephoned my Father on the Wednesday afternoon at 2.51 p.m. hoping that he would have woken up a little. He had. He was much better. I told him the dangers of morphine and asked him not to take any more. I told him that the drug would kill him if he continued with it. Apart from 'Goodbye, I love you dad,' my last words to him were: `If you take any more of that drug it will kill you.' They haunt me. But he wasn't very keen on hearing what I had so say. My dad could be incredibly patient. But when it came to medical matters he always wanted immediate solutions. When he started having a little prostate trouble I recommended that he try eating a handful of pumpkin seeds once a day. Twenty four hours after I made this suggestion he telephoned and rather grumpily told me that my suggestion hadn't worked. Sadly my dad believed that there was a pill for every problem. He liked pills. And GPs like prescribing them. When we cleared out my dad's house we filled one and a half black dustbin liners with bottles and packets of pills. I went once with him to see a specialist, shortly before his death, because he was finding it difficult to walk as far as he used to be able. `I can't walk uphill as fast as I could,' he said. `What are you going to do about it?' he demanded, staring rather belligerently at the consultant.

My dad agreed that the Oramorph made his breathing worse but said he liked it. He said he wanted to see documentary evidence showing that the drug was dangerous for patients in his condition. I said I would bring him the evidence the following day. My wife did a Web search that evening and printed out some suitable evidence to add to the textbooks I'd picked out.

I was telephoned at around 8.30 p.m. that evening (Wednesday 27th February) by the night nurse. She said my father was a bad colour and was having difficulty breathing. She admitted that he had been given another dose of morphine at 8.00 p.m. and told me that he had subsequently developed serious breathing problems. She told me that his condition had deteriorated alarmingly after he had been given the drug. I said I was planning to visit the following morning and repeated my request that he be given no more of the drug. I told her that in my view morphine would kill him. I said I would be in to see him the following day but hours later he was dead.

On my way down to Exmouth I received a telephone call from the nursing home to say that my dad had died.

Why wouldn't he listen to me and stop taking the drug? Simple. Some months earlier I had questioned another prescription which had been written for him. (After taking it he developed an irregular heart beat.) When my father had passed on my concerns to his doctor, the doctor had dismissed my worry; reportedly telling my father that, because I wasn't in practice, I was out of touch and out of date.

When I had seen my dad I asked to see the nursing home's drug records. The nurse I spoke to immediately said: `It's about the Oramorph isn't it?'

After a post-mortem a pathologist concluded that my father had died of his respiratory problem. There was a small amount of Oramorph left in his blood. Could the morphine have helped kill my father by exacerbating his respiratory problems? Would he have been alive today if he hadn't had that last dose? We will, of course never know any of the answers.

But the doctors at the hospital (where he had been for over two weeks) did not think he needed morphine (or, maybe, thought that it would not be safe for him to take it). The hospital did not regard him as terminal. (He was sent an outpatient appointment for March 13th). He did not complain that his pain had got worse after he had left the hospital. And he went from weak but relatively healthy to dead in less than 24 hours - after being given a drug which the manufacture states he should not have been given.

If he had needed a stronger painkiller why didn't the GP try a higher dose of the Fentanyl patch instead of prescribing morphine for an 87-year-old man with severe respiratory problems?

An article in *Pharmacology* advises that the most dangerous side effect of morphine is `respiratory depression'. *MIMS* magazine for doctors warns that the two first disorders listed as contradictions for Oramorph are respiratory depression and obstructive airways disease. All GPs receive, and should read, *MIMS*. And according to a leading medical website: `Respiratory depression (with morphine preparations) occurs more frequently in the elderly and debilitated patients, as well as in those suffering from conditions accompanied by hypoxia or hypercapnia when even moderate therapeutic doses may dangerously decrease pulmonary ventilation'. The West Midland Ambulance Service has warned that Oramorph should not be given to patients with respiratory depression or inadequate tidal volume. Oramorph, like all drugs, is particularly likely to be potent when given to elderly patients. Older patients tend to respond more dramatically to drugs than younger ones.

In the end, I decided there was no point in attending Dr Earland's inquest because the coroner informed me that she had already decided (before the inquest) that Oramorph did not cause my father's death. She agreed to accept witnesses but suggested that they wouldn't make any difference to her decision. And she decided not to have witnesses whom I considered vital at the inquest. It seemed to me that if you don't ask the right people the right questions you aren't ever likely to come up with the right answers. I felt it had become the sort of inquest where Kafka would have felt at home.

It was suggested by the coroner that if I wanted justice I should take action in the civil courts. I didn't want damages. What good are damages? The idea of suing in the civil courts reduced my father's death to the level of a faulty ladder on an uneven pavement. I was, I confess, reminded of Conan Doyle's remark that `some of these country coroners do think they are tin pot gods'. Conan Doyle was, of course, himself a doctor. He knew of which he spoke. A coroner is a medium level state functionary but one who has a great deal of power over his or her tiny domain, like a local VAT inspector, or a traffic warden. I found the whole inquest experience cold, unhelpful and traumatic. I've had friendlier encounters with HMRC. The whole thing was managed with all the subtlety and compassion of an MOT test. I didn't understand why the inquest wasn't being held in front of a jury. According to the leaflet I was given at the start of the proceedings, inquests are held with a jury: `if further deaths may occur in similar circumstances'. This was clearly the case in my father's death. My father's GP has not admitted that the drug was prescribed inappropriately and has, presumably, not changed his prescribing practices. Other doctors may well be prescribing the drug under similarly inappropriate circumstances. Ergo, there should have been a jury. There wasn't.

On 3.00 p.m. on 20th August 2008 I met a policeman, the coroner's representative, at a police station in Devon. He told me that the impression was that I was a bit of a nutter, that the coroner was aiming for `natural causes' and that the death was not taken very seriously because my dad was 87-years-old when he died. He said none of the other witnesses had been interviewed and weren't likely to be. We talked for some time. I explained exactly what had happened and he agreed with me that it would perhaps be surprising if the coroner didn't agree with me that the Oramorph was probably the cause of my father's death and that negligence was involved. `If he'd been a young child things might have been different,' said the policeman. 'The feeling is that your dad was old and had a long life so what are you going on about?'

I felt his theory explained the curious nature of the coroner who didn't bark. You don't get many rights these days if you're old.

Eventually, after it finally became clear that the coroner had already decided that the Oramorph had nothing to do with my father's death. I sent her this letter:

'When I started this long and tiring journey I hoped for two things: justice for my father (in the hope, perhaps, of a simple acknowledgement that an error had been made) and an opportunity to prevent the same thing happening again. The second of these was actually the most important. Nothing can change the fact of my father's death. But it is now abundantly clear that neither objective will be reached. More people will die in exactly the same way as my father died and the judicial system is not going to prevent this happening. What a missed opportunity! There was, here, a clear opportunity to warn doctors of the danger of prescribing inappropriate drugs (particularly to the elderly) with a specific example illustrating the consequences.

Your list of witnesses is disappointing, to say the least. I can think of two specific individuals from the nursing home who should be there. A senior member of staff agreed with me that Oramorph was making my father ill and agreed with me that the drug would kill him and that he should have no more of it. In addition, the nurse who gave the final dose would be able to describe my father's reaction to the drug and to tell us the time of his death. We know the time he was certified dead but I certainly don't know the time of his death.

On 7th August you wrote and told me that you intended to call the nurse who `allegedly agreed with you that Oramorph was seriously affecting your father's condition' and `the nurse who was on duty when your father died'. But your list now merely includes `a representative from the Cranford Nursing Home'. That could be an *administrator. Both the relevant nurses are easily identified and, presumably, traced.*

In addition you have no expert representative from the drug company which warns doctors not to give Oramorph to patients with my father's condition.

My lack of faith in your inquest is increased by the knowledge that you have, quite inexplicably in my view, already decided (before the inquest) that the drug which I am quite certain killed my father played no part in his death. (`Oramorph does not feature as the cause of your father's death' - your letter dated 7th August 2009.) The drug company insists that Oramorph should never be given to patients with my father's condition. (In my experience drug companies do not usually limit their market without good reason.) The theoretical medical evidence suggests that a normal dose of the drug could kill him. Hospital doctors refused to give him a similar drug just days beforehand. The clinical evidence shows that the first dose of the drug affected him adversely. And yet somehow you `know' that the final dose of the drug, inappropriately prescribed, did not kill him. I have studied the pathologist's report but I still have no idea how you reached this conclusion.

I would now like to withdraw from the process completely so that I can, at last, begin to mourn and to remember my father rather than fighting over the manner of his death. It has been enormously stressful to see a close relative killed by an inappropriately prescribed drug and to be denied anything remotely resembling proper justice.'

I did not know then how the coroner came to her conclusion. I still do not know.

I made a formal complaint to the General Medical Council (GMC) about Dr Hallmark and Dr Livingston. To my astonishment the GMC agreed with my father's GPs that any contradiction for the use of Oramorph in COPD patients is relative rather than absolute. They apparently ignored the fact that the drug company which makes Oramorph has an absolute ban on the use of the drug with

COPD patients. The drug company stated that Oramorph is contraindicated in any patients with obstructive airways disease. I asked the GMC to explain why the defending GPs' views were considered more relevant than the manufacturer's advice. They refused to answer. And they refused to consider evidence from the professional witnesses who observed the effect the Oramorph had on my father.

If I was astonished by that judgement I was utterly dumbstruck by the GMC's decision that it is acceptable practice for GPs to advise patients living alone, and in excruciating chest pain, to be told to call their own ambulance and then just wait for the ambulance to arrive.

That's medical care in Britain in the 21st century.

And I think it stinks.

I wrote to the GMC saying that I wanted to complain about their decision. I said I wanted to make a formal complaint about the GMC and the two employees who decided that a clear contraindication to the prescribing of a drug is of no consequence. `Under the Freedom of Information Act, would you please let me have the names and qualifications of the two GMC employees who decided that it is perfectly acceptable for a doctor to ignore a drug company warning not to give a drug.'

I didn't hear from them again.

The hospital weakened my father. They were, if you like, the picadors. I believe the GP then did the matador's work by prescribing an unsuitable drug.

In the end, nothing happened. No one was disciplined. No one apologised. Nothing changed.

The hospital believe they did nothing wrong.

Two GPs claimed they did nothing wrong.

The coroner said no one did anything wrong.

The General Medical Council agreed that no one did anything wrong.

I wrote to the police but they didn't bother to respond to my letter.

But everything you have read is the truth. So, now you decide.

Remember: my dad was given a drug the manufacturer said he should not have been given. Within minutes his condition had deteriorated. He then recovered but was given another dose of the same drug. Within hours he was dead. Neither the coroner nor the GMC thought there was a link between the two events and neither made any attempt to investigate any relationship between the two.

If it had all happened to a child, an asylum seeker or the wife of a minister would the result have been the same? Does being white, male and over 80 diminish the significance of a death? The case seemed very simple to me. A doctor prescribed a banned drug. Abundant evidence shows that the drug made the patient ill. The patient died soon afterwards.

Why should you care? Because you could be next.

I have spent my entire medical career exposing the dishonesties and incompetences of doctors. There is, therefore, no little irony in the fact that I believe that incompetent doctors killed both my parents.

But the fact is I know that my parents were killed only because I know what to look for. I've described how and why they died, and how the system did its best to cover up what had happened, not to point a finger but to draw attention to the extent of institutionalised incompetence within the world of medicine.

This wasn't a case of a patient being given the wrong dose of a drug. It was a case of a patient being given an entirely inappropriate drug. No one has ever apologised, expressed remorse or regret or admitted they made a mistake. So, one has to assume, the same thing will happen again. And again. And again. Prescribed drugs are one of the top killers in Britain today. The wrong drug can kill a patient just as surely as a bullet. How many other deaths are officially dismissed as natural causes? Is this through incompetence or a lack of caring or is it deliberate policy? How many deaths which should be investigated are never reported to the coroner? How many coroners refuse to investigate such cases?

Just how big is the iceberg?

3. Iatrogenesis: The New Epidemic

Officially, the big three killers today are cancer, heart disease and stroke. Things are much the same in all developed countries. Cancer kills rather more than 150,000 people a year in the UK. Heart disease kills just under 100,000 a year and stroke kills just over 50,000. Smoking (which kills largely through cancer and heart disease) is reputed to kill around 100,000 people a year. (The official annual death rate in the UK is around 300,000 which rather suggests that someone in charge of Government statistics can't add up very well but some deaths are, of course, listed as having more than one cause.)

The `big three' killers are responsible for the vast majority of deaths. Infectious diseases, the next big group of killer problems, are responsible for relatively few deaths. However, these official figures are misleading for one simple reason: doctors, the people who write death certificates and who decide a patient's cause of death, rarely admit that they themselves are responsible for killing a patient. Not many doctors are prepared to write `Me' on the line that asks for `Cause of death'. And you can't really blame them. Doctors, just like car mechanics, plumbers, interior decorators and everyone else, hate admitting that they've made a mistake. Most, as the old joke goes, just prefer to bury them quietly and hope no one notices.

Iatrogenesis (medically induced illness) does not officially exist as a cause of death. But every doctor with more than half a brain knows that many of the patients listed as dying from `cancer' or `heart disease' or `stroke' or `pneumonia' (or whatever else) died not because of an uncontrollable, untreatable disease but because a doctor, or a group of doctors, working alone or together with a nurse, or an entire hospital, screwed up. However, doctors are in such denial that iatrogenesis is not an official (or even an unofficial) medical speciality. It's as though heart disease were not a recognised speciality. Through a toxic mixture of hubris and self-denial, doctors underestimate the incidence, significance and consequences of iatrogenesis and the dangers of overprescribing prescription drugs. Despite all the evidence that exists iatrogenesis remains officially unrecognised as a problem. Why? Simple. To recognise it would be economically and professionally inconvenient.

Nevertheless, medical journals do occasionally publish articles in which attempts are made to estimate the number of people killed by doctors. There are never any precise figures because doctors don't put themselves down on the death certificate as the cause of death. But objective assessments make it pretty clear that doctors are, without a doubt, a major cause of disease, injury and death. Doctors kill a thousand times more people than terrorists, murderers or criminals. Far, far more people are killed by doctors than die in road accidents or train or aeroplane crashes. Doctors kill people by doing the wrong thing, by not doing the right thing or by not doing anything. There are many ways to kill a patient by mistake. And as procedures become more complicated, and drugs become powerful, so the number of ways in which doctors kill patients grows, grows and grows. The quality of medical care is now so low that I seriously doubt if one in every two consultations results in treatment that is timely, well-chosen, efficacious and genuinely certain to do more harm than good.

To a certain extent, things have always been this way, of course. Doctors have always killed patients. Most of them don't do it on purpose. The number of Dr Harold Shipmans around is, thankfully, quite small. But a patient killed by a mistake is just as dead as a patient who has been deliberately killed.

What really should worry us all is that things are constantly getting worse.

They are getting worse for several reasons. One reason is, undoubtedly, that drugs are more powerful and procedures more complicated. But the main reason that they are getting worse is that doctors are becoming increasingly incompetent.

The big question is, of course, how many patients do doctors actually kill? How many patients end up in coffins instead of going home because doctors screwed up?

Difficult question.

But I can guarantee one thing: it's far, far more than you thought it was. Doctors kill far more people than even the most pessimistic observer would imagine. Doctors are now a major cause of illness and death. Study the statistics and it becomes clear that throughout the `civilised' world doctors are right up there alongside heart disease and cancer as the big-time killers of the 21st century. A study in Australia showed that 470,000 Australian men, women and children are admitted to hospital every year because they have been made ill by doctors. The figures also show that every year 280,000 patients who are admitted to hospital suffer a temporary disability as a result of their health care. Around 50,000 of these suffer permanent disabilities. A staggering 18,000 Australians die annually as a result of medical errors, drug toxicity, surgical errors and general medical mismanagement. What a terrible indictment of the medical profession.

In America, the official death rate from medical `accidents' is running at around 200,000 a year. When doctors from the Harvard School of Public Health studied what happened to more than 30,000 patents admitted to acute care hospitals in New York they found that nearly 4% of them suffered unintended injuries in the course of their treatment and that 14% of the patients died of their injuries. This survey concluded that nearly 200,000 people die each year in America as a result of medical accidents. This means that more than four times as many people officially die from injuries caused by doctors as die in road accidents. I believe the real figure is probably considerably higher than this and there can be little doubt that many of the injuries and deaths are caused by simple, straightforward incompetence rather than bad luck or unforseen complications.

Figures in Europe are no better. In my book *Betrayal of Trust* I revealed that one in six British patients in hospital is receiving treatment because he or she has been made ill by doctors. Unfortunately, there are no official figures for the number of people killed by British doctors. Doctors in the UK don't accept that they ever make mistakes. (Although when I was last invited onto a radio programme to talk about the fact that one in six patients in hospital are there because doctors have made them ill, a doctor representing the medical establishment came into the studio to defend his profession and argued that patients could take comfort from the fact that the figures showed that five out of six hospital patients were *not* sick because they had been made ill by doctors.)

Coronary bypass operations are immensely popular among heart surgeons (and extremely profitable) but a major study conducted in Europe showed that many patients who don't have surgery live longer than those who do. Twenty years ago, American surgeons performed 350,000 coronary bypass operations and charged $14 billion for them. When one researcher studied 300 patients who'd had bypass operations at several hospitals in California he discovered that 14% of the patients would have thrived as well without surgery as with it while another 30% were borderline. Around 50% of lower back disc operations and up to 70% of hysterectomies are probably unnecessary. In America the death toll from unnecessary surgery alone has been estimated to be as high as 80,000 patients per year.

Around half of all the `adverse effects' associated with doctors are clearly and readily preventable and are usually a result of ignorance or incompetence or a mixture of both. The rest would be preventable with a little care and thought (and some better research).

Most people recognise the damage that other doctors can do but like to think that their doctor is an honourable exception. This is entirely understandable. After all, we all like to think that our relationship with our own doctor is special and that we have chosen someone reliable and knowledgeable to look after us. We like to think of our doctor as a personal and family friend. We all need to put some trust in the health care professionals upon whom we rely when we are ill.

But it is just as dangerous to assume that your doctor is entirely safe, sensible, knowledgeable, competent and error free as it would be to assume that you do not need to take care when driving, on the spurious grounds that road accidents only ever affect other people.

The underlying problem is that even good, kind, conscientious doctors - who are honest and honourable, who care about their work and who do their very best for their patients - can still make people ill. And can still kill people.

It has always been diagnostic skills which have differentiated between the good doctor and the bad doctor. Treating sick people is easy. If you are a doctor and you know what is wrong with your patient you can look up the correct treatment in two minutes. It's diagnosis that is difficult and since the days of cupping and leeches it has been diagnostic skills which have differentiated between the good doctor and the bad doctor. Sadly, doctors have handed that particular art over to machinery - with disastrous results. Modern doctors are now useless at making diagnoses. Young, newly trained doctors are the worst - partly it is true because they are inexperienced, but mainly because they have been trained to rely on tests and investigations rather than on developing their own diagnostic skills. One in four cancer cases is missed simply because doctors don't know what to look for, don't know what questions to ask and don't listen when patients hand them clues that should really start alarm bells ringing. It's hardly surprising that more and more patients are described as having a 'mystery illness'.

All this is terrifying.

For if the doctor doesn't make the right diagnosis then it doesn't matter how many wonderful drugs he has at his disposal.

When researchers examined the medical records of 100 dead patients who had been shown by post-mortem to have had heart attacks they found that only 53% of the heart attacks had been diagnosed. What makes this even more alarming is the fact that half the patients had been looked after by experts in heart disease. A study across 32 hospitals which compared the diagnoses doctors had made when treating 1,800 patients with the diagnoses made after the patients had died (and could be examined more thoroughly) showed that doctors had an error rate of nearly 20%. When 80 doctors were asked to examine silicone models of female breasts they could only find half the hidden lumps. That's a 50% failure rate even though the doctors knew that they were being tested and observed. Another study showed that doctors had missed diagnoses in dying patients up to a quarter of the time. Experts concluded that one in ten patients who had died would have lived if the correct diagnosis had been made. Yet another group of researchers revealed that in two thirds of patients who had died, important, previously undiagnosed conditions were discovered in the post-mortem room. A report published after pathologists had performed 400 post-mortem examinations showed that in more than half the cases the wrong diagnosis had been made. The authors of this report said that potentially treatable pathology was missed in 13% of patients; that 65 out of 134 cases of pneumonia had gone undetected and that out of 51 patients who had suffered heart attacks doctors had failed to diagnose the problem in 18 cases. Some years ago it was estimated that inexperienced doctors working in casualty units killed at least one thousand patients a year. Now that doctors are even less experienced, and even more poorly trained, I suspect that the figure is far, far higher than that.

When it comes to disorders of the mind (the big growth industry of the 21st century) doctors are even more incompetent. A study of 131 randomly selected psychiatric patients showed that approximately three quarters (75%) of the patients had probably been wrongly diagnosed. (It is always difficult to be precise about mistakes in psychiatry because it isn't a science at all.) In many cases patients are diagnosed as having - and are then treated for - serious psychiatric problems when their symptoms are caused by drugs they have been given for physical problems. Whole wards full of patients have been diagnosed, treated and classified as schizophrenic when in fact they were suffering from side effects produced by the drugs they had been given by prescription happy doctors. The idea that anyone would describe psychiatry as a science is utterly absurd. Nothing that psychiatrists claim as `fact' can be proved by any means recognised by scientists; there are no proper controls and if an experiment is repeated it rarely produces the same result. The ultimate absurdity is the fact that psychiatrists claim that only they are fit to judge the effectiveness of their recommendations. Psychiatry is black magic masquerading as science.

The result of the fact that the psychiatric profession has sold itself to the pharmaceutical industry is that patients are now often treated for conditions that sane people would not regard as illnesses. Patients who feel guilty, worried, or concerned about the state of the world are likely to find themselves labelled and drugged for life. Those who are too timid, too reserved, too kind (a condition now regarded as akin to weakness) too gullible or too anything are likely to find themselves filled to the gills with some poisonous but enormously profitable concoction. Psychiatrists never suggest that patients might live with their symptoms, or (heaven forbid) find some non-pharmacological solution. There is never any discussion of side effects or any suggestion that the long-term consequences of therapy might turn out to be worse than the long-term consequences of the disorder. Psychiatrists and drug companies have been so successful in convincing politicians of the effectiveness of their so-called `speciality' that virtually all the money available for the care of mental patients is now spent on pills (even though there is invariably no evidence to show that they do any good at all). Institutions caring for the mental ill were closed down (using the excuse that they were politically incorrect) and the patients who needed care were dumped into the community, to wander the streets. It's difficult to blame drug companies for this sad state of affairs (they exist, after all, solely to make money) but it's easy to blame psychiatrists.

The sad truth is that psychiatry is the greatest con on earth. Psychiatrists and general practitioners have become increasingly enthusiastic about drug therapy in recent decades. They claim that they can treat a wide range of disorders with psychotropic drugs and so a goodly portion of the nation now regularly gulps down happy tablets. The result is that the incidence of mental health problems is increasing. Officially, one in two people in Britain is incurably mentally ill. (Despite this the number of beds available for mental health patients is constantly shrinking. This is, of course, because the mentally ill make an ineffective lobby.)

Psychiatry isn't a science at all and it isn't even an art. It's more of a confidence trick; a collegiate confidence trick with pretensions of grandeur. The simple fact is that there is no evidence that there is any such thing as `chemical imbalance'. Ask any psychiatrist about this and he will agree that `chemical imbalance' is a still unproven theory. It's never even been properly tested so how could it ever be proven? So how can psychiatrists and drug companies possibly treat the problems which they claim are caused by `chemical imbalance'? The bald truth is that psychiatry is no more a science than witchcraft. It is a perfect example of pseudoscience running riot. Cinema legend Samuel Goldwyn was right when he said that anybody who goes to see a psychiatrist ought to have his head examined. A big part of the problem lies in the fact that modern medical thinking is based upon the Cartesian principle that the mind and the body can be treated separately. The modern clinician still does not see the mind and the body as a single unit (that is why orthodox practitioners don't believe in holistic medicine) and this leaves the way open for psychiatrists to play around with the human mind.

You may be surprised to learn that psychotropic drugs (widely promoted by doctors who have close links with the companies making them) have no provable, useful effects. They do, on the other hand, have massive and provably serious bad effects (such as death). How are these drugs supposed to work? That's not exactly known. It is, however, known that they flatten the emotions and cause a numbing and dullness of the mind which make patients taking the drugs less aware of their problems. Patients become so numb that they don't notice the nasty world around them. These drugs don't cure mental symptoms; they simply cover them up. The best patients can hope for is that the side effects aren't too bad. And the damned psychiatrists are constantly finding new excuses to prescribe (and to add to drug company profits). So, for example, they even prescribe drugs for people who are shy. They call it `Social Anxiety Disorder' and there is a powerful drug for it, with appropriately powerful side effects. There are drugs for all shades of neuroticism. Heaven knows what sort of future mankind has when you remember that all great art and all great inventions were the result of neurotic minds.

Psychiatrists have a rapidly growing dictionary of labels which they can apply to their patients. The big problem with their labels (I'm talking about diseases such as ADHD and schizophrenia) is that none of these diseases (none) actually exists. Not in the way that pneumonia and tuberculosis exist, with real signs and symptoms. Psychiatric disorders are created and agreed upon by groups of psychiatrists who meet together and think up new disorders. I'm not making this up. There is proof that diabetes exists. There is scientific evidence to show that heart disease is real. But there is no proof to show that any psychiatric disorders really exist. They are labels which are often created merely to find a market for a newly invented drug. Diagnoses are made, and treatment begun, without any evidence that a patient has anything wrong that can be treated. Drugs are prescribed in the vague hope that they will produce an improvement. Most of the time they produce a change - but the change is more likely to be a deterioration than an improvement.

A vast variety of entirely non-existent diseases is becoming forever commoner, taking up a constantly increasing part of a constantly decreasing health service budget. Many psychiatrists claim (apparently meaning it) that we are *all* mentally ill and that we *all* need treatment. This is not a social comment so much as an excuse to hand out prescription drugs which do more harm than good. (My own experience of medical colleagues who are psychiatrists is that they are all barking. The Brazilian psychiatrist who shot a patient because `they all come in here and just want to think about themselves, no one thinks about *me*' wasn't that exceptional. Psychiatrists are pretty screwed up people; deviants and neurotics. That's why they become psychiatrists. All the psychiatrists I've known have been as mad as hatters. I suspect that they became psychiatrists because they couldn't deal with the logical science of real medicine. They chose, instead, to drift into the world of psychiatry where nothing is written down in black and white, and where judgements are made subjectively rather than objectively.

Many psychiatrists have such close links with drug companies that they promote drug therapy for all with missionary zeal. Whenever psychiatrists make a suggestion one only has to ask `Who benefits?' to see what is going on. In 2010 a proposal to screen the entire population of Britain for depression was abandoned, possibly because it was realised that a virtually bankrupt nation could not afford to conduct an inefficient but incredibly expensive survey into mental health, possibly because a civil servant somewhere realised that the cost of providing anti-depressants would push the nation further into bankruptcy and possibly because someone realised that the nation was so despairing that a survey would probably show that the whole country was depressed. (That, I am sure, was the plan. Just think of the profits to be made out of prescribing antidepressants for everyone in the country.)

Drug companies concentrate on me-too drugs, the moneymakers, ignoring diseases that affect the Third World and ignoring rare diseases. They want long-term medications for long-term problems and psychiatric drugs are the most profitable. Drug companies love mental illnesses. Patients don't die from them. They live long, healthy lives and so, once diagnosed, can be given drugs for decades. Patients never get better and so the drug therapy is eternal. These disorders are self-reinforcing. When told they are `mentally ill' people tend to become anxious, introspective, less interested in the outside world and more self-obsessed. Doctors talk about exogenous and endogenous depressions but the only real difference between the two is that in one the cause has been found and in the other it hasn't. The two varieties of depression are basically identical. Both are caused by stress.

So much money is spent on utterly worthless psychotropic drugs that there isn't any money left for the long-stay hospitals that the vulnerable and the unstable desperately need. Community care doesn't work, and everyone knows it doesn't work, but it's cheap. Very cheap. The NHS has dumped thousands of mentally ill patients on the streets. It has also put a huge and intolerable burden on the families of the chronically sick. Sad though it may be there will always be some people who need to live permanently in institutions and who benefit from attending workshops and properly run day centres. The State has abandoned the mentally ill because they don't vote as a group, don't employ lobbyists, don't have support from television celebrities and aren't considered photogenic.

The sad truth is psychiatry is a nonsensical speciality. And all its treatments are unproven rubbish. Aversion therapy, behaviour therapy and hormonal rebalancing are nonsense. Drug therapy is as dangerous, in its way, as psychosurgery. Diagnoses are made without evidence existing. Treatment is prescribed in a purely subjective way. And the diagnostic symptomology is so vague and far reaching that I could, without much difficulty, find some definable mental illness in every person in the UK.

Some people make friends when they travel. I have an acquaintance who can't pop into the local supermarket without finding new chums to add to his formidable Christmas card mailing list. If he goes for a walk in a deserted park he will somehow come back with half a dozen new pals. I'm not good at making friends. Too shy, I suppose. But this means that I am suffering from quite a number of mental disorders. According to the official definitions and symptom lists I reckon I am suffering from autism, ADHD, ODD, obsessive compulsive disorder and several dozen other psychiatric disorders. And I don't mind betting that you are too. Today, just about every human emotion or behavioural pattern is a psychiatric disease; an official medical diagnoses. Shyness, homesickness, suspicion, having ups and downs and distractibility are all diseases. There are special drugs for all these disorders. New diseases soon likely to be classified include: `apathy disorder', `compulsive shopping disorder and `Internet addiction disorder'. If your doctor says you have one of these then you're officially mentally ill. Lack of self control and impatience are now officially recognised as diseases. Welcome to the worldwide club. There's a drug with your name on it. And a long-term sick note just a scrawl away. Many of the new diseases relate to children. There's a good reason for this. Once a child is started on a drug there are likely to be decades of prescribing (and profits) ahead.

How do psychiatrists define new diseases? Easy. A bunch of 27 of them (most of them with links to drug companies) simply decide what is officially a disease. Psychiatrists actually have meetings to vote on whether diseases exist or not. Homosexuality used to be a disease, but political correctness pressures resulted in a vote deciding it was not. That's what psychiatrists call `science'. Thanks to their efforts, everyone can be diagnosed as mentally ill and everyone diagnosed will be treated. Providing drugs for mental illness is an industry worth a third of a trillion dollars a year. It's hardly surprising that new mental diseases come thick and fast. There is no evidence that any of the drugs prescribed can `cure' anything (partly because none of the diseases being treated can be properly diagnosed or specifically identified) but there is plenty of evidence showing that the drugs being used produce a huge variety of known, and sometimes deadly, side effects.

There are now nearly 400 psychiatric medical diagnoses in the official lists. There are specialists and drugs for all these diagnoses. And not one of the 400 has been tested or proven to exist. If you ever have a dull moment in your life get yourself a copy of the latest edition of the *Diagnostic and Statistical Manual of Mental Disorders* and flick through it looking for the daftest diseases. It's hardly surprising that no one is now truly normal. These diseases aren't found in a laboratory or identified by epidemiological studies: they are created in marketing departments. And why not? Drug companies can make 500,000% profit on the drugs they sell.

Psychiatrists, apparently blind to what is going on around them, seem deliberately unaware that we live in a society where toxic stress is endemic and the human consequences inevitable. 'Our contemporary Western society, in spite of its material, intellectual and political progress, is increasingly less conducive to mental health, and tends to undermine the inner security, happiness, reason and the capacity for life in the individual,' wrote Dr Erich Fromm. 'It tends to turn him into an automaton who pays for his human failure with increasing mental sickness, and with despair hidden under a frantic drive for work and so-called pleasure.'

Drug companies use marketing experts to persuade well people they are ill and need to take a pill, preferably permanently. Patients' groups are set up and funded. In the UK, one of the big groups catering to autism sufferers takes drug company money. Journalists are bought and diseases created. In the business this is called disease mongering. It's big business. Research is funded by drug companies and not surprisingly, the research with embarrassing or inconvenient results never gets published. Medical journals (which rely on drug company advertising) are often bent as are journalists. The medical community is corrupt and up to its eyes in drug company money. When TV programmes want to speak to a doctor about drugs they invariably contact one of the 'hired hands' recommended by the drug companies. Doctors who tell the truth are banned and marginalised. Governments say they can't find any doctors without conflict of interest to sit on committees assessing drugs. (Well, I'm here. An acknowledged expert on drugs and iatrogenesis and a licensed, registered medical practitioner. But, surprise, surprise, they never approach me.) Doctors go to conferences run and or paid for by drug companies. No doctor who is likely to oppose or question drug therapy will be invited to speak. (The last time I was invited to speak to NHS personnel I was quickly uninvited when my name was spotted on the list of speakers.)

Many of the commonest problems are behavioural conditions associated with children. These are diagnosed subjectively and can increasingly be diagnosed by nurses and teachers rather than by psychiatrists. The doctors are too busy signing the prescriptions to bother with actually seeing patients. ADHD, autism and Asperger's syndrome will all become default conditions soon. Their incidence is increasing so absurdly fast that children without one of these conditions will be regarded as abnormal and will, of course, need treatment. Autism became popular because it's a damned sight more convenient for drug companies to create a new disease than it is to accept that children can be brain damaged by vaccines (another drug company product). For drug companies it is a double whammy. They avoid the vaccine lawsuits. And the new diagnosis enables them to sell treatments for a newly created and non-existent disease. Parents are often enthusiastic and don't seem to care that the evidence shows that a walk in a park is better than drugs for children with ADHD. Pushy, expectant parents with not very bright children temper their disappointment by accepting that their children have a new and fashionable disorder. A doctor's note showing that a child has ADHD enables him and family to jump to the front of the queue at theme parks, and to jump the queue for school lunch. It's hardly surprising that one in 20 in Britain has ADHD. And yet the symptoms are so vague that I doubt if there is a child in Britain who doesn't have it. The more intelligent doctors who prescribe drugs for ADHD and other entirely imaginary diseases know damned well that the whole thing is a scam: useless products for imaginary disorders; non-existent solutions for non-existent problems. I suspect that many patients know its emperor's new clothes stuff; the intelligent ones anyway. They go along with the con because it is easier to accept (and to tell their friends and relatives) that their child is rude and badly behaved because he has a brain disease, rather than because he is, well, rude and badly behaved. And poorly brought up. And they get extras too. Sympathy, care, even extra money. A disabled sticker for the car. No need ever to wait in queues. Only the stupidest doctors, together with social workers and school teachers of course, are unaware that it is all a scam; an expensive, dangerous but massively profitable scam.

New diseases are being invented almost daily. There's another exciting disease around now. It's ODD (Opposition Defiant Disorder). The symptoms are an absence of respect for authority and anger management issues. Those with ODD are surly, defiant, uncooperative and hostile towards authority figures. Psychiatrists believe that ODD affects between 1% and 16% of all school age children (nice of them to be so precise).

I've no doubt that many of these children need help. But some need help to deal with real problems (deafness, low IQ etc.) and most need help to deal with the overwhelming stress and pressure in their lives.

I can't prove my theory. But they can't prove any of theirs either. And I have two advantages. First, my theory is not based on commercial expediency. I profit not at all from it. The psychiatric profession cannot say the same. Second, I am prepared to match my track record at spotting dishonesties and medical trickery against that of any ten psychiatrists the medical profession wishes to offer.

So, what the hell is really going on? Is all this just about profits?

Well, here's an interesting quote from the National Association for Mental Health: `Principles of mental health cannot be successfully furthered in any society unless there is progressive acceptance of the concept of world citizenship. World citizenship can be widely extended among all peoples through applications of the principles of mental health.'

And here's a quote from Dr G Brock Chisholm, psychiatrist and co-founder of the World Federation of Mental Health: `To achieve world Government, it is necessary to remove from the minds of men their individualism, loyalty to family traditions, national patriotism and religious dogmas.'

Ah yes, of course.

The bottom line, of course, is that since the psychiatrists and the drug companies decide what mental illness is and is not, the incidence of mental illnesses will continue to soar. The lunatics have truly taken over the asylum. Psychiatry enables doctors to offer specific solutions (and treatments) for all the symptoms and signs they cannot explain any other way. It isn't patients who are the nutters, it is the doctors, nurses and administrators who believe this mumbo jumbo.

No one ever does anything about any of this. The incidence of iatrogenesis is the fastest growing problem in healthcare but most members of the medical establishment deny that it exists and the rest just close their eyes and hope that no one notices. Everything is going to get worse before it gets better.

Modern medical education is often lamentable and frequently appalling - with lecturers too often teaching medical students about organs and tissues rather than living patients. Students are taught plenty of facts but very little vision. They are given directives but never directed. The whole programme seems designed to test a student's ability to memorise information (some of it easy to look up and much of it purely arcane and irrelevant in 99.99% of real life) instead of teaching students how to develop their instincts and their innate healing skills. Modern medical education is dangerously narrow and unimaginative; designed and managed by people who are so deep inside the establishment that they might as well be living on Mars (or Venus). The real world, the real lives of patients, the real problems people face are all dismissed or ignored. The problem starts at secondary school, of course. The target culture has encouraged schools which are keen to stand high on the list of successful establishments to persuade pupils to take GCSEs in easy subjects such as `media studies', `food technology, `outdoor pursuits', sports leadership' and so on rather than proper, crucial subjects such as English (Language or Literature), mathematics, a foreign language, history or geography. Children leave school with a handful of irrelevant and entirely useless qualifications and a less than rudimentary education. Never before has a country produced so many students with so many qualifications and so little learning. A diploma in horse care is officially ranked as equivalent to four good GCSEs. A diploma in hairdressing is officially worth six good GCSEs. Schools churn out illiterates and innumerates as though they were in demand. I have, for many years, received a huge amount of mail and it is possible to tell the age of correspondents not by the shaky handwriting of the octogenarians but by the quality of writing and spelling. When these children end up cutting hair, writing writs or running Government departments their illiteracy is of little consequence but for doctors-to-be it is vital that they know how to read and to understand the meaning (and hidden meaning) of what they read. It is the low level of starting education which is at least partly responsible for the low standards of medicine practised by young doctors today.

Today, medicine attracts the half-hearted, the half-witted and the half-interested. Medical schools don't teach knowledge (though they think they do, and certainly like to give the impression that they do); instead, they teach prejudice and propaganda and black magic and they at best studiously avoid, or at worst positively forbid, the study of evidence outside the mainstream which shows, for example, that serious heart disease can be most effectively treated without drugs or surgery and that the placebo effect is crucial to the effectiveness of the doctor patient relationship.

Students are not taught that judgement isn't derived solely from numbers and graphs and charts and laboratory results. They aren't told that judgement is a combination of conclusions drawn from evidence; it is derived from instinct and intuition as much as learning and knowledge.

Modern medicine has become focused on narrow issues and doctors are not taught or encouraged to study the alternatives (both those within and those without orthodox medicine) and to then assess the options wisely and with an open mind.

Inspiration is an essential part of creativity but modern doctors are trained to exclude inspiration and therefore to exclude creativity. Students are 'protected' from anyone who doesn't toe the drug company party line. These restrictions mean that today's doctors can only make diagnoses by rote. That's a fundamental problem with medical education. Medical schools suppress imagination and creativity. The establishment crashes down heavily on anyone willing to question authority or to disobey the rules. And the further a student goes within the system the stronger these restrictions (these failings) become.

Doctors have become obedient, unquestioning tools of the establishment; accepting information and advice as though it were factually based, and merrily prescribing whatever junk they are told to prescribe. Doctors are controlled by bureaucrats so they think and behave like bureaucrats. The vast majority of modern doctors have no instinct, no intuition, no inspiration, no courage, no truth, no dignity, no common sense and no passion. The profession has created a generation of doctors who are quite incapable of thinking for themselves and who have been beaten into intellectual and ethical submission by a medical system which is controlled by a grotesque mixture of drug companies, politicians, spiritually and ethically dead doctors, and bureaucrats who regard patients as a damned nuisance. Most doctors are trained to be incapable of original thought and incapable of lateral thinking. They follow the pre-determined system and plod their way through their caseloads without ever thinking for themselves.

The ability to work, and to learn, is a talent as much as any other and all the great medical thinkers have been hard workers. They didn't spend their days filling in their forms or attending meetings with bureaucrats or social workers. They had ideas, tried them out and learned. That doesn't, and cannot, happen today. It is not surprising that young doctors find it difficult to make decisions. You can teach the science of medicine but you can't teach the art, the instinct, the passion or the dedication. These have to be discovered through time and by being nurturing. Today, there is no time and no nurturing. Today's doctors are not bright enough or creative enough or imaginative enough to have doubts and without doubts you are lost. Modern doctors spend far less time in training than their predecessors. New rules and regulations limiting the amount of time doctors can spend working mean that the modern consultant or general practitioner will be put in a position of responsibility when still relatively inexperienced. At schools everywhere the reliance on multiple choice tests (which can be marked by computer and therefore liberate teachers and allow them to enjoy their hobbies) has destroyed imagination, initiative and literacy.

Another problem is that the Internet has encouraged cheating among students. For example, 234 candidates attempting to study medicine all wrote that their passion for the subject had been sparked after: `burning a hole in my pyjamas at age eight with a chemist set' and 166 began with: `For as long as I can remember, I have been interested in...'. Around 275 applicants to become nurses all started their applications with the words: `Nursing is a very challenging and demanding career.'

When students learn deceit at an early age they will fit easily and quickly into the deceitful world that medicine has become.

(Incidentally, the Internet is now such an unreliable source of information that innocent and naive webusers become over-loaded with misinterpretations, hand me down prejudices and ready made, fit anyone preconceptions.)

Sadly, the ignorance didn't just start with the Internet. Not all that long ago a study of GPs reported in a medical newspaper showed that a quarter of general practitioners did not know about the connection between smoking and heart disease while, amazingly, a fifth of GPs were unaware that cigarettes could cause lung cancer. (One magazine editor refused to publish an article I wrote quoting this survey on the grounds that he couldn't believe that doctors could be so ignorant).

But although older doctors have their faults it is the younger doctors who frighten me most. Today, students are desensitised to horror long before they become doctors. They have been exposed to years of watching violence on television, on DVDs and in games (and although there is a watershed which ensures which children are supposed to be protected from the sight of naked breasts on their television screens they are still exposed to endless hours of violence in taxpayer subsidised programmes such as Eastenders).

Moreover, young doctors do not listen to their own voices. They do not know they have voices of their own. They do not even know they are entitled to voices. They do not know that they are entitled to think for themselves. It is hardly surprising that doctors behave like sheep (though without the natural charm of those gentle herbivores) and stick to the party line, whatever the party line might be, without ever questioning a word of what they are told. Like good civil servants (which modern State-employed doctors assuredly are) they are trustworthy Statists; marching to the party tune and never wavering in their support for their inglorious leaders.

The current generation of medical students learn little and read little. They don't learn how to think critically or creatively or to reason out problems for themselves. They have very poor general knowledge and no interest in or knowledge of their patients' lives and so they miss all sorts of diagnostic clues. It is hardly surprising that young doctors find it difficult to make decisions. They are trained to respond to the rules, the whole rules and nothing but the rules.

Modern doctors are taught to make decisions by computer rather than by experience or intelligence or intuition. Actually, come to think of it, modern doctors behave like rather second rate computers. They feed themselves facts and test results and then spew out answers without regard for the sense they are making.

The best doctor I ever knew didn't even know how to read an X-ray report let alone an X-ray and when he wasn't feeling too well he would still do his home visits but he would stand in the downstairs hall and shout questions to the patient in bed. His advantage was that he knew his patients. He visited them at home and saw how and where they lived. He talked to them about their work. He knew their families. He lived within the community. Medicine is a lot easier when you understand a little about people.

That good doctor, whom I remember with fondness, knew that a good doctor needs an open mind, an ability to hear between the lines and an ability to read a silence; an ability to put a patient at ease, to mask the real questions, and sometimes to ask the really important questions as an apparently half relevant afterthought.

He knew that doctors can sometimes diagnose without listening to the words, just the music that comes through is enough. And the silences. The pain in a man's eyes and in his voice, the way he holds his body; all these things speak volumes. A good doctor needs soft eyes and an ever-open heart.

Those are lost skills.

Studies have always shown that doctors are at their worst when dealing with patients with whom they feel uncomfortable. Narrow training means that doctors feel uncomfortable with a wide range of people. They often have difficulty relating to, talking to or acquiring information from people of `different' races, sexes or social backgrounds to their own. But the biggest problem is surely the fact that modern doctors are taught to rely almost entirely on technology and are rarely encouraged to build up any communication skills of their own.

Old-fashioned doctors used to rely on what their patients told them and on what their eyes, ears, noses and fingertips told them. Most important of all, perhaps, was the sixth sense that doctors used to acquire through years of clinical experience.

Modern doctors rely too much upon equipment which is often faulty, frequently badly calibrated and more often than not downright misleading. For example, nearly every published study on the subject puts the error rate for doctors reading X-rays at between 20% and 40%. Radiologists working at a big hospital disagreed on the interpretation of chest radiographs as much as 56% of the time. And there were potentially significant errors in 41% of their reports. Even when X-rays are read for a second time only about a third of the initial errors are spotted.

Another problem is that the vast majority of students never learn how to do research or judge published research. This is largely because the vast majority of doctors, and nearly all university lecturers, don't know how to do it either. Medical schoolteachers should teach cynicism and have a special course in iatrogenesis. The first is frowned upon and most doctors have never even heard of iatrogenesis - even though it is, along with circulatory disease and cancer, one of the big three killers.

All this is rather depressing.

But in life it is important to know what we are up against. If you're going to survive to a good age - and stay healthy - then you need to know something about doctors. Many people are prepared to put all their trust in doctors. That can be a dangerous mistake. Doctors now do more harm than good. They can - and do - save lives. But they kill a lot of people too.

There is nothing new in the fact that doctors kill people. Doctors have always made mistakes and there have always been patients who have died as a result of medical ignorance or incompetence.

But, since we now spend more on health care than ever before, and since the medical profession is apparently more scientific and better equipped than ever before, there is a savage irony in the fact that we have now reached the point where, on balance, well-meaning doctors in general practice and highly-trained, well-equipped specialists working in hospitals do more harm than good.

The epidemic of iatrogenic disease which has always scarred medical practice has been steadily getting worse and today most of us would, most of the time, be better off without a medical profession. Most developed countries now spend around 8% of their gross national products on health care (the Americans spend considerably more - around 12-14%) but through a mixture of ignorance, incompetence, prejudice, dishonesty, laziness, paternalism and misplaced trust, doctors are killing more people than they are saving and they are causing more illness and more discomfort than they are alleviating. Most developed countries now spend around 1% of their annual income on prescription drugs and doctors have more knowledge and greater access to powerful treatments than ever before, but there has probably never been another time in history when doctors have done more harm than they do today.

The bottom line is that doctors are, with cancer and heart disease, one of the three biggest killers today. And doctors don't just kill people. They also maim and injure and disable. Most people don't see what is happening, of course. They don't realise how often doctors miss diagnoses, or make the wrong diagnoses. If you aren't medically qualified you won't see exactly what is going on. The inescapable conclusion is that patients should learn to be sceptical about the medical profession. Just about everyone I know who has seen a doctor in the last 20 years has been mistreated. Most of the patients didn't have the faintest idea how badly they had been treated.

I constantly receive a barrage of case histories of incompetence and cover-ups. A friend today described how his father died after a liver biopsy was performed while he was a day patient. Unbelievably, my reader's father was taking prescribed aspirin to thin his blood but no doctor told him to stop the aspirin before the biopsy. The man went into hospital as a day patient but when he left he went to the morgue, not to his home. Doctors should have a Government health warning stamped on their foreheads. `Beware: This Doctor May Harm Your Health'.

In this hard new world we are all of us at risk. A few years ago I nearly lost a kidney as a result of medical incompetence. Two radiologists who had looked at X-rays of my kidneys told me that I had kidney cancer. They gave me the names of two local surgeons and suggested that I choose one. (When I asked for more information about the two surgeons I was told, very helpfully, that one had a good bedside manner while the other was competent.) I insisted on a scan and a third opinion. I was then told that my slightly misshapen kidney was a perfectly normal variation. The third radiologist showed me a textbook illustration which showed precisely why the other two radiologists had been wrong. If I hadn't had the third opinion I would have lost a perfectly healthy kidney and undergone totally unnecessary major surgery.

Death by medicine has become the default condition; State sanctioned, legal, and professionally approved homicide.

4. The Triangle Of Evil

Doctors, hospitals and drug companies constantly claim that the modern medical profession has, during the last century or so, dramatically improved life expectation. The increasing size of our elderly (and disabled) population is, say the industry's supporters, a direct consequence of medical progress.

This is a monstrous lie. It's a lie so big that it would make politicians blush.

Looked at superficially the statistics seem to support this claim. It is, for example, undeniable that there are more 70, 80 and 90-year-olds around now than there were a century ago. The idea that doctors have pretty well conquered illness and are helping us defy death itself is a warm, comforting one. But it's a fraud. A great big lie worthy of the most devious politician. The medical profession and the drug companies are guilty of a confidence trick of gargantuan proportions.

When the medical profession, together with the pharmaceutical industry, claims that it is the advances in medicine which are responsible for the fact that life expectancy figures have risen in the last one hundred years or so they are being either inestimably stupid or egregiously dishonest.

Figures for the UK are difficult to get hold of because the British Government traditionally regards every health care statistic as a State secret, to be shared only with the pharmaceutical industry, but figures published by the United States Bureau of Census show that 33% of people born in 1907 could expect to live to the age of 7

5. Later figures show that 33% of the people born in 1977 could expect to live to the age of 80. Remove the improvements produced by better living conditions, cleaner water supplies, and the reduction in deaths during or just after childbirth and it becomes clear that doctors, drug companies and hospitals cannot possibly have had any useful effect on life expectancy. Indeed, the figures show that there has been an *increase* in mortality rates among the middle aged and a *dramatic increase* in the incidence of disorders such as diabetes, arthritis, heart disease and cancer.

The truth is that the inventor of the flush lavatory has saved a million times more lives than any doctor. It is not the men who discovered antibiotics - and who now prescribe them with such reckless overenthusiasm - whom we should thank for the virtual disappearance of some of the best known killer infectious diseases of the 19th century but the men who dug our sewers and laid the first water pipes. Improved sanitation facilities have meant that the number of babies dying - and the number of women dying in childbirth - has fallen dramatically. For adults, life expectation has not been rising. You can prove this to yourself quite simply by checking the ages at which people died a century or two ago. Look in history books or local graveyards and you will see that although many babies and children died young the average lifespan was often 70 or 80 years. Despite all the expensive razzmatazz of modern medicine life expectation has simply not increased in the last century or so. The biblical promise of three score years and ten has been fairly steady for centuries.

The evidence shows that the apparent improvement in life expectancy which has occurred in the last hundred years is not related to developments in the medical profession or to the growth of the international drug industry. If doctors really did help people stay alive then you might expect to find that the countries which had most doctors would have the best life expectation figures. But that isn't the case at all. Moreover, look at what happens when doctors betray their principles, embrace mammon, go on strike and leave patients to cope without professional medical help. You might imagine that without doctors people would be dying like flies in autumn. You'd be wrong; dead wrong. When doctors in Israel went on strike for a month admissions to hospital dropped by 85% with only the most urgent cases being admitted, but despite this the death rate in Israel dropped by 50% - the largest drop since the previous doctors' strike 20 years earlier - to its lowest ever recorded level. Much the same thing has happened wherever doctors have gone on strike. In Bogota, Colombia doctors went on strike for 52 days and there was a 35% fall in the mortality rate. In Los Angeles a doctors' strike resulted in an 18% reduction in the death rate. During the strike there were 60% fewer operations in 17 major hospitals. At the end of the strike the death rate went back up to normal. And I am told that when hospitals and clinics were closed down by terrorists in Sri Lanka the Registrar General reported that the number of reported deaths had fallen. Whatever statistics are consulted, whatever evidence is examined, the conclusion has to be the same. Doctors are a hazard rather than an asset to any community.

The incidence of diabetes, for example, is now reported to be doubling every ten years and the incidence of serious heart disease among young men is increasing rapidly. Today, death rates from heart disease among adults are 50 times higher than they were at the start of the century. Bacteria are becoming increasingly resistant to antibiotics and the number of disabled and incapable citizens in developed countries is increasing so rapidly that it is now clear that, as I pointed out in my book *The Health Scandal*, the disabled and incapable will, by the year 2020, outnumber the healthy and able bodied.

The fact that there are more old people around these days has nothing to do with drug companies and doctors providing us with better medical care (as doctors and drug companies claim) but is a result of several factors things.

First, the population is bigger.

When the population is greater the chances are that there will be more old people. There are more old people living in London than there are old people living in Ross on Wye because there are more people living in London than there are people living in Ross on Wye.

Unbelievably, doctors and drug companies ignore this simple statistical fact.

Second, infant mortality is much lower today than it was a few decades ago. In England in 1900, one in four children didn't reach their 11th birthday. Many died as babies. Others died in childhood. Today less than one in 100 children fails to reach their 11th birthday. And, as a result, life expectation seems to have improved dramatically. This isn't difficult to explain. Imagine you have a family consisting of four people. One dies at the age of three. One dies at the age of 97. One dies at 30. And the fourth dies at 70. The four individuals have lived to 200 between them. Their average lifespan is 50 years. Now assume that the child who died at the age of three lives to 103. That will push up the average lifespan to 75 years. A century or so ago many newborn babies never saw their first birthday. They were killed, largely, by infectious diseases. Cholera, smallpox and typhoid killed millions. The big change that has taken place has involved not doctors but better sewage facilities, cleaner water supplies, more spacious homes, more food and better built towns and cities. All these things have helped slash infant mortality rates.

And so people *seem* to be living longer.

Today, there are more old people around because less are dying as infants. And, of course, as the population grows so the number of old people increases.

Next, there has for many decades been a steady reduction in the number of children being born in the developed world. Terrified by what was originally described as the birth explosion time bomb millions of couples decided to limit the size of their families - or not to have children at all. The development and introduction of the contraceptive pill and of sterilisation techniques for both men and women made this easy. In contrast this has definitely not been the case in the developing world and the global political consequences are far reaching. In Muslim countries birth rates are extremely high and the average age in those populations is inevitably much younger. A society which is predominantly composed of young, healthy individuals obviously has a very different outlook to a society which is dominated by older, often unhealthy individuals. The future is Muslim. Our ageing, Western, largely Christian society has very little future.

Moreover, the incidence of disability among the elderly has been increasing steadily too. Today's elderly are nowhere near as fit as their ancestors were. Our fat and toxin rich diet is just one factor which has led to a steady increase in the incidence of cancer, obesity, heart disease, arthritis and many other causes of long-term disability. Mental illness such as chronic anxiety and depression, caused by the unavoidable `toxic stresses' created by the structured society in which we live, are now endemic - as are the myriad illnesses caused by the powerful drugs frequently prescribed by doctors with such carelessness.

The drug industry and the medical profession are guilty of creating a new version of the post hoc ergo propter hoc fallacy. (Because B happened after A then B was caused by A.) Doctors and drug company executives argue that adults live healthier lives (a lie) and live longer (another lie) because of developments made by the drug industry. It would be just as reasonable if the shoe industry claimed that people live healthier lives, and live longer, because of developments made in the shoe industry.

In reality, the evidence shows not that doctors and drug companies are saving a vast number of lives but that the modern medical profession has become a danger. Indeed, the person most likely to kill you is your doctor. Modern, Western doctors, equipped with fancy drugs, exotic forms of surgery and impressive sounding radiotherapy techniques, are ranked alongside cancer, heart disease and stroke as major killers.

Four out of ten patients who are given drugs suffer serious and sometimes potentially lethal side effects. If the drug you're prescribed is going to save your life that's probably an acceptable risk. But how many patients who are merely suffering from something annoying or uncomfortable would willingly take a drug if they knew it might kill them? There are hugely profitable drugs on the market which have never saved any lives but which have killed or made ill countless thousands of people.

One in six patients in hospital in Britain is there only because he has been made ill by doctors. Most are suffering from unpleasant or downright dangerous drug side effects. In America, bad reactions to legal drugs kill far more people annually than all illegal drug use combined.

You won't hear any of this from most doctors, of course. Doctors are notoriously reluctant to admit that the treatments they recommend can do harm. There are several reasons for this.

First, they often don't know how dangerous drugs and other treatments can be. In just about every Westernised country in the world doctors receive most of their post graduate education through meetings and journals which are sponsored by drug companies. And drug companies don't spend too much of their time warning doctors about drug side effects. Global drug companies don't exist to find cures or help people: they exist solely to make money.

Second, doctors are frightened of being sued.

Third, there are nearly half a million clinical research papers published every week. No doctor on the planet can read them all - or even have the faintest idea what warnings they might give. Useful reports are lost among the irrelevant, commercially inspired dross. Any evidence showing that doctors and drug companies are killing people is easily overlooked or allowed to slip behind a convenient filing cabinet.

Finally, the natural human unwillingness to admit responsibility is exceptionally well developed among doctors who often think of themselves as having god-like qualities. Admitting to mistakes reminds doctors that they are human and fallible.

The bottom line is that during the last century, doctors and drug companies have become louder, more aggressive, a good deal richer and far more powerful but life expectancy has not risen as a result of any of their activities. Together with politicians (and the States they represent) they have become the triangle of evil.

5. State Run Medicine Doesn't Work (The NHS Was A Terribly Stupid Idea)

The NHS was founded on a dangerous series of myths and misconceptions.

Aneurin Bevan, the politician who founded the NHS in 1948, did so on the basis of a local insurance group which provided health care in return for weekly contributions. He was a keen fan of Karl Marx and the best we can say for him is that he probably meant well. (Winston Churchill wasn't so kind. He once described Bevan as a squalid nuisance.) Unfortunately, Bevan clearly didn't understand that you can't turn a small, amateurish, honest little organisation into a huge, national organisation without exchanging the passion, the purpose and the goodwill for an enormous amount of harmful bureaucracy.

Bevan seems to have believed that a national health service was a `good thing' because he felt that health care, like education, should be free to the user. He wanted the State to be responsible for paying all the bills; installing the State machinery between doctors and patients. That was his first absurd, calamitous mistake. Why should the State provide a free health care service? The notion that health care or education should be `free' because they are essential is downright silly. It would make far more sense to say that water and shelter should be free. Why is it a sign of a caring society to have free health care and free education? It is argued that these are essentials for life and so must be available to all without cost. This argument can be destroyed in one word. Food. I don't see anyone offering free food to everyone - regardless of need. It is far better to give poor people the money to buy whatever food they need than to give them State controlled food hampers. No one suggests that supermarkets should be run by the State and food made available to anyone who wants to wander in and wheel a trolley. And yet it would make more sense to have nationalised supermarkets than it did to nationalise health care.

Besides, most of the NHS is not essential to life (infertility operations, breast enlargement and sex change operations are hardly vital to survival) and most of our education system is not crucial (the bit that teaches media studies springs to mind as an example of the utterly unnecessary). Am I the only one to think it odd that we provide patients with free infertility treatment but charge patients for essential dental treatment, for spectacles and for drugs they need to stay alive. Too much of the NHS is organised to satisfy the doctors rather than the patients. Home deliveries have more or less gone for pregnant women. Home visiting has been reduced to a bare minimum. There are waiting lists to see a consultant, to have basic tests done and to get into hospital. People even have to wait to get an appointment to see their GP. Family doctors now hide behind duty rostas, deputising services and white-coated receptionists. Cottage hospitals have been replaced with huge, bug-ridden, expensively equipped battery hospitals. It should be no surprise that the British were never healthier than they were during the Second World War. The death rate of workmen over 50 years of age has for some years now been higher now than it was in the 1930s. More people than ever are dying of heart disease and the evidence shows that a man or woman who has a heart attack will probably be better off staying at home than going into hospital. We have more doctors than ever but much of their postgraduate education is paid for by the drug industry and, as a result, more than half the adult population and over a third of our children take a drug every day of their lives. Britain leads the world in fertility treatment and yet thousands of mentally handicapped patients roam the streets because the NHS provides no facilities for them. Four out of five patients who go to see the doctor have nothing wrong with them that wouldn't get better with a good holiday, a modest win on the pools or a little friendship and understanding. People want guidance, support, kindness and caring but thanks to the Bevan's health service they get drugs and a system that doesn't give a damn.

The idea that hospitals and doctors should be part of some national system is nonsensical. Bigger simply means employing more bureaucrats. The existence of a central authority, and the employment of layer upon layer of administration, makes the NHS expensive and inefficient.

Bevan's other, incredibly stupid, idea was that the NHS would help eradicate illness. Really. It apparently never occurred to him that some people might like going to the doctor, especially if someone else was paying for it.

Nor did he realise that the NHS would end up approximately four times as expensive as private care because of all the administration.

And, most important of all, in my view, he completely failed to understand that the NHS would destroy the traditional relationship between patient and doctor (employer and employee) and create a new one (supplicant and civil servant bureaucrat, dispenser of good things and keeper of the gate). He also failed to understand that anything Governments organise is required to be inefficient, uncaring and incompetently run.

Bevan believed that the NHS would pretty well cure all illness. The opposite turned out to be true. Knowing nothing about medicine and even less about people he thought the cost of the NHS would fall as people were cured. In fact he produced an extraordinarily expensive and wasteful bureaucracy which is addicted to spending. If he had wanted to help the poor he should have set up a scheme to give money to the poor so that they could buy private health care. This would have been cheaper and more efficient but most importantly it would have maintained the purity of the relationship between doctors and patients. The NHS encourages a paternalism that is stifling and destructive. Doctors, not patients, take decisions. Medical decisions are designed to conform more to the wishes and needs of the doctor than the patient. Putting the legs of a pregnant woman into stirrups is for the convenience of the doctor not the patient. Too often patients allow decisions to be made for them. Few doctors are prepared to allow patients to live with mild disabilities. For example, a patient who gets mild chest pain after walking for five miles will be told that he needs surgery. A patient who develops leg pain after cycling for a few miles will be referred to a surgeon. No doctor will today think of telling a patient that he can, if he wishes, simply live with his symptoms, adapt his life to live around them, and change his lifestyle to produce a permanent improvement. Doctors make the decisions on how much pain is tolerable and on when life is worth living. These are ethical decisions, value judgements and moral pronouncements. The NHS encourages medical imperialism.

Today, the big question that no one ever dares to ask is: 'Is the NHS a good thing?'

As questions go it is the herd of rampaging wildebeest in the sluice room. Politicians, journalists and earnest members of the medical establishment talk endlessly about restructuring and reorganising the NHS. But they never talk about getting rid of it. No one with the authority to do anything ever dares question the effectiveness and efficiency of the NHS. No one ever asks if it is necessary. No one ever questions whether it is providing patients with the best type of health care. No one ever questions the role of the State in providing health care. No one ever dares ask whether the NHS is good value for money. The NHS has become a political icon. It is inconceivable that any politician would dare to suggest a debate to discuss shutting it down.

And, in my view, most important of all, no one dares to discuss the ways in which the NHS has damaged the relationship between doctors and nurses on the one hand and patients on the other.

For me the big problem with the NHS is not simply the fact that it is enormously wasteful and bureaucratic (though it is both of those things) but the fact that it has produced a fundamental change in the all important relationship between health care professionals, on the one hand, and patients, on the other. There is no dignity. There is no respect. There is no pride.

Because they work for the State, doctors and nurses are now civil servants. GPs have attempted to retain their independence by officially remaining self-employed. But it's an accounting independence not a primary independence, designed more to minimise personal tax liabilities rather than anything else. GPs claim that they are self-employed but it is more of a tax fiddle than a serious ideological claim. For all practical purposes GPs, like hospital staff, are civil servants in the same sort of bracket as tax inspectors, planning officers and Home Office officials. And, like all civil servants, they enjoy vast amounts of authority and very little responsibility.

The fundamental problem with civil servants is that their loyalty is to the State, rather than to the people who are paying their wages. Civil servants tend to acquire a superiority complex. They absorb the power they represent and become incredibly snotty when dealing with `members of the public'. (Just try dealing with a tax inspector or a traffic warden if you doubt me.) Whenever I go into a Post Office I am reminded that there is a huge difference between Government employees and other people. Government employees don't care; they don't have any interest or pride in what they do. They turn up for work because it's marginally more interesting and much better paid than staying at home and watching daytime television. That's how the NHS now operates. Doctors and nurses really don't give a toss whether you live or die as long as they get home on time.

The standard Government employee knows that what he does doesn't really matter - as long as he is loyal to the State. Incompetence and laziness are excusable and will be defended by the State and its other apparatchiks. The State's employees know that they must always defend anything done on behalf of the State because if they don't the State's authority will be diminished. And as far as the State is concerned, authority is everything. Ronald Reagan, former President of the United States of America, was spot on when he said that: 'The most terrifying words in the English language are: `I'm from the Government and I'm here to help.'

This may not matter terribly much when we're just dealing with tax inspectors. But it does matter a good deal when health care professionals are involved. When health care is involved, the standard State employee mentality is simply unacceptably dangerous.

There are a host of problems with having a State-owned and run health service. Decisions made by Governments are bad because they are always made for the wrong reasons. And in the world of medicine the wrong decisions are made for the wrong reasons by the wrong people because there is no one to stop them. The right people (those few doctors and nurses who care) are bullied, frightened and overwhelmed. The truth isn't just ignored, it is hidden and suppressed. Those who dare to ask inconvenient questions are silenced. It is crucial to remember that anything the State organises is organised for the benefit of the State. That's the way statism works. As Ayn Rand wrote: `The difference between a welfare state and a totalitarian state is a matter of time.' Large corporations are organised for their own benefit and have identities, purposes and aims of their own. And any organisation set up by the State will exist to protect and preserve its own integrity and status.

Everything is made worse because the three parts of the unholy trinity (the Government, the drug industry and the medical profession) all support one another and deliberately work against the interests of the patients.

In the days before the NHS, doctors offered cut-rate or free services to patients who couldn't afford to pay. I once looked through the accounts book of a doctor who worked in the 1920s and 1930s. He charged his well-off patients a fee for every consultation or home visit. But if he knew that patients couldn't afford his fees he charged them half-price. And if he knew that patients couldn't afford even that then he waived his fee and charged them nothing. Hospitals and hospital consultants did the same. The medical profession did not include doctors who would allow their patients to die for lack of treatment. No one was turned away because they did not have the money to pay for a consultant or a bottle of medicine. Doctors considered that they had a responsibility towards the less fortunate. Free medical care was widely available for the poor.

It is perhaps difficult to accept that such a system can work. We have been brainwashed into thinking that the State must take responsibility for everything. But this has happened simply because those who work for the State want to control everything; they want to extend their power into every aspect of our lives. We have lost the ability to imagine a system wherein free people might solve problems without threatening one another with lawsuits or threats of violence - as our society deals with problems.

The traditional relationship between doctor and patient was simple. The patient asked the doctor for help. The doctor offered advice and treatment. The patient paid the doctor. No one else was involved. (Things were different in China where patients paid their doctor when they were well and stopped paying when they fell ill but this doesn't really concern us and nor does it affect my argument.) If the doctor wasn't much good his patients didn't go back to him. The doctor (and nurse) had a vested interest in providing patients with the best possible care.

The introduction of third parties into this relationship (in the form of the State or an insurance company) changed the dynamic of the relationship in a fundamental way and changed the responsibility and loyalty of the doctor.

The bottom line is that patients need control over doctors and the best way to arrange this is for them to have control over the money (even if the State has to give them money to spend). As St Matthew warned us: `No man can serve two masters.'

Today, doctors have lost all their independence. They are paid by the State and so their primary allegiance is to the State. The traditional, basic link has been broken and the doctor is responsible to the State and not to the patient. This is why doctors vaccinate their patients even though the evidence clearly shows that it's a dangerous and ineffective business which benefits only the vaccine manufacturer (and, to a certain extent) the State. Doctors have become obedient and fearful and are bullied by the bureaucrats. Moreover, medical staff will in future be increasingly constrained and instructed by meddling, ignorant, self-interested, self-elected lobbyists representing a myriad patients groups, clinical networks, health and well-being boards; by citizens' panels; by official and unofficial busy bodies and by the now usual plethora of health and safety morons.

Doctors used to be primarily concerned with protecting and serving their patients. Today, they are primarily concerned with protecting their relationship with the State and, like most civil servants, serving the State and making as much money as they can. Authority corrupts as much as power. And the medical profession is now part of an authoritative system which is utterly corrupt. The State machine is demanding, and it demands blindness of its servants; blindness to anything new and potentially threatening or critical of its systems and methods. Purpose and value have been abandoned. Doctors are bribed with money and the promise of less work. The machine destroys but rewards generously. State-controlled health services lead to a confused mixture of needs, wants and demands with lobbyists and politicians deciding how the money should be spent. The open-ended demands on the NHS's obviously limited resources are never met and so choices have to be made. Some live and some die. The strongest lobbyists win. The weakest patients die.

The whole organisation of the NHS is devised to satisfy the State's requirements, rather than the needs or best interests of patients. Doctors are supposed to serve patients but they are constantly ordered around by State bureaucrats. They do what the State tells them to do because the State is the master. So, for example, when the NHS becomes involved in GP care it promotes larger medical centres because these fit more comfortably into the bureaucracy. The State forces GPs to adopt appointment systems (which are unpopular with doctors and patients and which have been proven not to work well) because the State likes control.

Separating the interests of doctors and patients, and forcing doctors to identify with and become allies of the State (their employer) has meant that the triumvirate, the unholy medical trinity of doctors, drug companies and State, has become united and has created what is effectively a single organisation. The losers can only be patients. The normal counterbalance to a special interest monopoly, such as the unholy trinity created by doctors, drug companies and Government, is the existence of a powerful body with other interests but patients as a group are too weak and too ill-informed (and inevitably too frightened when they do take an interest) to protect themselves. They need support, help, independent, honest advice and guidance. All those things used to come from doctors but the balance was changed when the NHS was created and it has been getting worse throughout the NHS's existence. Today, policies which might benefit patients are forgotten while policies which benefit the unholy trinity are pursued zealously, selfishly and without feeling or compassion. When the hospital in Budleigh Salterton wanted throw my mother out of her bed, her then GP, who might have been expected to speak on her behalf, spoke with the hospital. The State employees stick together to defend the interests of the State. The trinity campaigns vociferously, buys the best lobbyists and creates laws to control those who oppose it. It also controls the media because journalists and editors have no choice but to believe what doctors tell them to believe. Dissidents are silenced even within the profession. The trinity controls everything and buys all the power it needs. The trinity either convinces the public or confuses it so that clear thinking and sensible, objective conclusions are impossible to reach. Doctors as State employees are afraid to make decisions in case they make the wrong decisions, so they go by the book; they follow the test results and they hire committees and consultants to produce reports and recommendations which are invariably so vague that there can be no blame if things go badly.

Because NHS staff are Government employees they have high job security. Self-interest is controllable in companies and businesses because consumers and shareholders do have *some* power. But Government employees are immune. They use the State to promote their self-interest at the cost of the taxpayers - in their case, patients. Of course, there are moral and honourable employees. But they are overwhelmed by the system and just as a chain is as strong as its weakest link so everything depends upon the selfishness of the most selfish employee. We have to remember that the NHS is one of the world's largest employers and the good tend to be overwhelmed and exploited and dispirited by the bad, who are not above using threats to get their own way. Government departments, such as the NHS, have no concept of loyalty or service because they don't have to rely on customers paying their bills and coming back. Apologies are never made because the State is never wrong.

The NHS spends money in the wrong areas. It has, like many large Statist organisations, become concerned primarily with its own survival, and more concerned with the protection and enrichment of its servants, than with looking after the people it is supposed to look after.

The NHS is a great organisation for doctors, nurses and bureaucrats. But it is disastrously expensive for the State. And it is terrible for patients. Doctors and nurses go through the motions but they are now civil servants and civil servants always look after themselves and the State before they look after anyone else. Inevitably, this means that patients come last. Patients are regarded as something of a nuisance because hospitals and health centres would run much more efficiently and comfortably without them. Like other State employees, doctors and nurses are overpaid and underworked. The NHS was always a naive and appalling idea. The Government cannot run anything efficiently. They certainly cannot and should not run health care.

Because of the State's intervention (and the absence of any link between money and work), doctors working for the NHS are now grotesquely overpaid and underworked and demanding (their union, the British Medical Association, was the first to protest when a Government report pointed out what everyone has known for years, that public sector workers don't pay enough for the pensions they get). Within the NHS (as with all other State departments) money has been separated from effort. With the usual disastrous consequences. Genuinely caring, sensitive young people don't want to go into medicine because it has become overregulated and controlled and bureaucratic. People who like money, filling in forms and obeying authority will flock to medical schools. But those people will make terrible doctors. There is no integrity within the modern NHS. Medicine today is all about money. Doctors may tell what they think is the truth but they don't tell the whole truth because they don't know the whole truth; they just tell the part that the drug industry doesn't mind being told. And, we must always remember, Governments can never be trusted. The diagnosis of cancer of the lung was virtually forbidden in France for many years because the Government held a monopoly over the sale of tobacco.

The sole aim of the NHS is to provide secure, undemanding employment for large numbers of people. The NHS is the third largest employer in the world and the aim of the modern NHS is not to cure or to care for patients but to provide employment for a vast army of jobsworths, many of whom earn six figure salaries and are provided with pension funds worth millions of pounds. The success of the NHS is measured not by the number of patients it helps (or at what cost) but by the number of artificial and dangerously irrelevant targets it meets. One significant result of this is that in a curious and amazing way the NHS encourages the under-treatment of some patients and the over-treatment of others.

Doctors and nurses are members of the world's primary service industry but in Britain the NHS has encouraged them to serve themselves above all others; it is a culture of selfishness that precludes caring. Patients are regarded by bureaucrats, doctors and nurses as at best an inconvenience and at worst a nuisance. Everyone working for the NHS seems to have forgotten why they are there. Separating consumer from cheque writing just doesn't work in an era of selfishness. There is no such thing as `public service' these days.

Within any large healthcare organisation, patients would be well advised to start each medical experience with the notion that everyone they meet is an idiot who cares only about their paycheque and getting home early. Patients may meet a few well-meaning folk, and a tiny few who really care, but, in order to protect themselves, and to give themselves the best chance of survival, patients should no more expect to meet sensitive, undemanding, caring people working in a hospital than they would expect to find caring, sensitive souls working in a tax office or car showroom. It may be an unpleasant and depressing thought but it is inescapably true that the people you meet in any State-run organisation are there because they are paid to be there. Forget all historic notions of vocation and dedication. And remember: anyone who works for the NHS is a Government employee.

Whenever State medical systems have been created they have proved to be a mistake. Statist politicians in other countries drool over the NHS and claim that it is a success. But they only claim it is a success because they are told it is a success and because they want it to be a success. If they looked at it closely they would realise that it is a failure. The truth about the medical system the rest of the world is told is wonderful, and wants to emulate, is that it kills people at great expense.

The NHS has proved only too vividly that the Government really has no place in health care. A Government controlled health service is unhealthy for everyone. The State way is to take all the authority and the responsibility away from people. And that is, in the end, disastrous. Patients have been taught to become totally dependent on the system and more aware of their rights than of their responsibilities. By deliberately and systematically taking over responsibility for our health, and by ignoring the fact that in the majority of illnesses the body can heal itself, NHS doctors have increased the demand for resources and they have produced a new type of medical problem: doctor-induced illness in patients who never needed treatment in the first place. The 21st century craze for interventionism is slowly killing us. In the 19th century health care was long on charity and short on science. Today, health care is long on science but short, woefully short, on charity and understanding.

And things have been made infinitely worse by the fact that political changes have put enormous pressure on a poorly designed health service. Now that Britain is part of the European superstate, and run by the European Union's meddling bureaucrats, the nation no longer has any control over the number of people allowed into the country. This is a problem because the Government has not built up enough infrastructure to cope with all the immigrants. The overpopulated UK is in crisis and, now that former Prime Minister Brown has wrecked the economy for generations to come, the infrastructure will never be repaired or brought up to standard to cope with the people who are flooding in. (The only good thing is that the level of immigration will soon stop because, thanks to EU distributions, countries such as Poland and Romania are improving rapidly and will soon be more prosperous than the United Kingdom and will offer better health service facilities.)

The real tragedy is that no one in politics (or the medical establishment) will ever dare question the usefulness or purpose of the NHS. Institutional cowardice means that politicians will refuse even to consider the possibility of closing down what has become a dangerous, administrative nightmare. And sheer professional greed and self-interest mean that doctors (who know they would never make as much money if they were in private practice) will never campaign for the abolition of the golden goose. Instead of fighting against the system on behalf of their patients, doctors now *are* the system. Doctors and nurses have become institutionalised. They are part of the State. They have been bought, indoctrinated and incorporated into the bureaucracy. And the tragedy is compounded by the fact that patients have been isolated by that same system.

Doctors and nurses are now making big money out of the Government. They fight for their own pay and conditions of service but they no longer fight for the patients they are paid (and obliged) to serve.

Britain has an increasingly incompetent, increasingly expensive and decreasingly trustworthy infrastructure. Britons can no longer trust the police to keep the streets safe. Britons are abused by loutish border guards if they dare to leave the country. Britons are treated as criminals by the clerks working for HMRC. And the main purpose of the NHS is now to provide wealth, security and a leisurely existence for the vast army of lazy, self-centred ruffians who work for it.

Doctors and nurses accept everything and question nothing. They have sold their souls to the State. There are much better ways to provide free health care than by allowing the State to run things.

Medicine is now owned and controlled by politicians and drug companies and bureaucrats. They make the rules and pull the strings and although it is taxpayers who pay the piper it is the corporate string-pullers who choose the tunes. Doctors and nurses are not on *our* side. They are on *their* side. Too many are now officious and spiteful; beholden to the rules. And it is all happening everywhere in the world. Medicine is becoming increasingly institutionalised and State controlled. The evil trinity (State, medical profession and drug industry) has gone global.

6. How Hospital Staff Have Betrayed Patients

Over recent years there have been shocking and systematic failures of hospital care in NHS hospitals, with patients routinely neglected, humiliated and left in pain. Thousands of patients have died as a result of poor treatment. One independent enquiry documented cases where patients had been left unwashed for up to a month and left without food, drink and medical treatment. The conclusion was that managers had been `preoccupied with cost-cutting, targets and processes' and had lost sight of their basic responsibilities. Astonishingly, none of the responsible managers responsible has been taken to court. (Doctors and nurses have professional responsibilities. Administrators, who have all the authority, have no professional responsibilities and apparently no accountability.)

I have little doubt that in all the hospitals where patients have been dying unnecessarily the staff (including doctors and nurses) convinced themselves that they were providing patients with excellent service. And, equally, I have no doubt that an enormous number of patients and relatives and hospital visitors must have ignored all these awful things and believed that the hospitals concerned were doing a wonderful job. It wouldn't surprise me in the slightest to hear that the managers responsible for all this pain, agony and death, have thick files of letters from patients and relatives thanking them for the excellent care. The truth is that neither patients nor relatives know precisely what to expect.

Walk into an NHS hospital and you will find demented patients in awful pain. You will find patients with terrible bedsores (the bedsore is a classic sign of bad nursing). You will find patients who are starving to death or dying of dehydration because the staff can't be bothered to feed them or give them fluids. You will see patients so dehydrated that their lips are bleeding and sore. You will see patients dumped in a chair, sitting in urine soaked incontinence pads which have clearly not been changed for hours. You will see obvious signs of malnutrition. These aren't patients in Third World countries. They aren't patients in badly run care homes. They are patients in major NHS hospitals. I know it is true because I have seen it time and time again with my eyes.

    Patients awaiting surgery are sent home because the hospital has run out of money and can't afford the sutures and other surgical equipment needed to operate on them. An 83-year-old woman with dementia was sent home from hospital in the middle of the night without her family being informed. The next day she was found dead, alone in her bedroom.

    A pregnant woman rang an NHS hospital to say that her baby was on the way and that she was coming in as planned. `There is no room,' said the hospital. `We are full.'

'What do I do?' asked the woman.

'Look in the yellow pages and find another hospital,' she was told.

Dirty sheets are reused in hospitals, just as they are in the dirtiest, cheapest, nastiest doss houses. But hospitals aren't supposed to be doss houses. They are places where the people in the beds are, by definition, all ill. Many of them with infectious diseases. I can understand bureaucrats accepting the re-use of dirty sheets. They are nasty, uncaring people. But doctors and nurses?

Dignity and respect are not words which the modern hospital employee understands. Not, at least, when applied to patients. Many hospitals still have mixed wards - with male and female patients forced to abandon their natural dignity in the interests of hospital economy (so that the administrators can take yet another huge pay rise). Governments repeatedly promise to make sure that mixed wards are done away with. Inevitably this promise is quickly forgotten and abandoned.

A generation or so ago most hospitals employed an almoner. It was her job (and the job was invariably held by a woman) to take care of patients' social problems. If an elderly patient was worried about the cat she'd left at home the almoner would find someone to feed it. If a woman worried that her children might need help the almoner would sort something out. If a patient was going home after a long stay in hospital the almoner would help ensure that the house was prepared. The almoner played a vital part in helping patients rest and recover.

Today, none of these things are done.

And yet our hospitals are awash with social workers who regard practical problems as beneath them and spend their days organising meetings to discuss meetings.

The result of all this is that NHS hospitals are best at dealing with mechanical, easy solvable, easily identifiable problems. If you have an uncomplicated broken leg then a hospital will probably be able to deal with it efficiently and relatively safely - as long as you manage to convalesce at home rather than on a hospital ward. With other, more complicated problems, however, hospitals can do a great deal more harm than good.

Back in the Middle Ages people were terrified to go into hospital. They knew it was a sentence of death. Relatives started digging your grave as you went through the doors of the local infirmary.

Things are getting that way in Britain today.

British hospitals are now among the worst in the world. One survey of NHS staff showed that only 44% thought that they would be happy with the standard of care provided if they were patients in their own hospital. Many British patients are now travelling half way round the world to get treatment in hospitals where patients are treated quickly, efficiently, hygienically and with respect. So, for example, hospitals in India are offering attractive package deals for British patients who can't wait two years for treatment or who don't fancy the idea of being killed by an antibiotic-resistant hospital infection. Officially, adverse drug reactions kill 18,000 people a year and cause 600,000 hospital admissions in the UK every year. In reality things are far, far worse than that.

It's called a National Health Service but it isn't. In 1971 I made a television programme for the BBC in which I explained that there were massive variations in the types of treatment available in different parts of the country. I used a blackboard, a long stick, a large map and several large sheets of paper to explain how treatments varied in different parts of the country. (This was, of course, long before the days of computer graphics.) There was, I claimed, no real `national' health service. Nothing has changed in principle although I suppose it is quite likely that there have been changes in the nature of the inequalities prevalent in the various regions. To call it a `National' Health Service is an absurdity that should merit investigation. Virtually the same programme (updated with fancy graphics) was broadcast while I was writing this book over a third of a century later.

One of the common arguments in favour of the NHS is that everyone gets the treatment they need without having to pay for it. This is, of course, a myth. Even allowing for the fact that some patients are denied treatment on the grounds of cost, and others are denied treatment simply because the area where they live does not offer the treatment they need, there is another big problem: NHS staff select patients for treatment on the basis of their perceived need and `value' to society.

Some readers may be shocked to know that the National Health Service already operates a selection system for treatment. But it has done so for many years. (English patients are particularly likely to be affected. Scottish hospitals have plenty of money; though it comes, of course, from English taxpayers.) When treatment is expensive it is provided for those patients who are regarded as the most deserving. And how does our system decide which patients are most deserving? Simple. A young married man with lots of children will be at the top of the list. An elderly man who lives alone will be right at the bottom of the list.

And so the NHS will provide life saving treatment for an unemployed scrounger of 36 who has a wife, a mistress and eight children. But a great, elderly painter or composer will be allowed to die.

Meanwhile, as people die for lack of resources, the NHS merrily spends more than Ł50 million a year on translators for patients who cannot speak English. The NHS provides translators for 160 languages including Cherokee and Cebuano. The fact that there are no registered users of those languages in Britain doesn't seem to concern the people with the cheque books.(Try visiting a hospital in Turkey or Greece and asking for a free translator.)

And is it not absurd, unfair and just plain wrong that NHS money is spent on providing couples with fertility treatment and women with breast enlargement operations while thousands of patients are dying because they have to wait weeks for essential, simple diagnostic X-rays? Surely, life saving should come first and life enhancing come second.

In military hospital units doctors operate a simple but effective system whereby those whose need is greatest get seen first. It's a sound principle. Life saving should come first and life enhancing should come second. But in the NHS the people who receive the best (and fastest) treatment are the patients who are represented by the most efficient lobbyists.

Today, well over twice as many people are killed in hospitals by infections as are killed on the roads. The reason? Filthy wards, unhygienic practices, scandalously poor cleaning, grubby operating theatres and staff who never wash their hands. There are more such infections in British hospitals than anywhere else in the world. Why? Simple. British hospitals are dirtier than hospitals anywhere else in the world. Why? The staff in British hospitals are the laziest and most incompetent hospital staff in the world.

If you live in Britain and have to go to hospital for any operation or procedure, you now have a 50% chance of getting a worse disease from being in the hospital. That's official. And if you do survive the experience and get to go home there is a good chance that you will leave malnourished. Staggeringly, one in five National Health Service (NHS) patients leaves hospital officially malnourished. Some patients don't eat because the food is inedible and looks unappetising. For others the taste and quality of the food is irrelevant; they stay hungry because no one helps them eat. Staff dump food on a patient's table and then collect it, untouched, half an hour later. The patient, starving hungry, hasn't eaten because he or she couldn't reach the food. Some are too weak or too disabled to feed themselves. Staff put food in front of semi-conscious patients and then walk away. In the 21st century NHS the patients slowly starve to death. One NHS patient who was blind couldn't see the food put before her. No one bothered to feed her. `It's not my job to feed the patients.' I've heard the staff say. Others simply state that they aren't allowed to touch patients or come into any sort of contact with them. And, of course, nurses now regard feeding patients as beneath their professional dignity. They are far too important to do such simple things. Other patients complain that the food they are given is shrink wrapped in impenetrable plastic. It's a sort of modern NHS torture. The patient can see the food but they can't get at it. It is the greatest indictment of our hospitals that patients actually die in them because they have not been given food or fluid. It was recently announced that in future nurses will be able to decide that a dying patient should not be resuscitated. Why not? Nurses in Britain already decide that patients should die by not being fed. Are they sadistic, or just stupid?

NHS hospitals are now so badly run, so filthy, so unprofessionally managed that they are good only at dealing with easily solvable, easily identifiable, mechanical problems. They can probably manage a broken arm without too much trouble. But when faced with anything more complicated they are likely to do more harm than good. The evidence has shown for years that patients who have heart attacks are better off staying at home than going in hospital. Anyone who goes into an NHS hospital for non-essential elective surgery should be refused treatment on the grounds that they are not mentally fit to sign a consent form. Hospitals have become unsuitable for the healthy - let alone the sick. In general, patients will survive for longer if they avoid the NHS. The survival rates in NHS institutions are awful. The standard of health care is among the worst in the world. Hospitals are run by people who don't give a damn about anything other than bonuses. Whether you are at home or in hospital it is, at night and weekends, easier to find a plumber prepared to come out than it is to find a doctor prepared to visit. An NHS manager in charge of the complaints system in a London hospital fell ill and needed treatment as an in-patient. He afterwards admitted that he 'got into difficulties finding out who was his doctor, what medicine to take and when he was getting out'. What a bloody country. What a bloody NHS. What a bloody disgrace. People in Britain pay to go into private hospitals not because they expect to be treated more kindly, or because they expect better medical treatment, but because they hope that they will not be allowed to die from starvation or thirst and they believe, probably correctly, that the wards will be cleaner. It is, perhaps, hardly surprising that the people who run (and work for) the National Health Service, prefer not to use it. Civil servants working at the Department of Health are entitled to be members of the Benendeen Healthcare Society which serves one million British Telecom, Post office and civil service workers. If they fall ill they get to go to a luxury private hospital. Most people working in the NHS admit that if they (or a member of their family) falls ill they would not want to be treated in the hospital where they work. I will repeat that. Most people working in the NHS admit that if they (or a member of their family) falls ill they would not want to be treated in the hospital where they work. (The NHS used to ask staff members if they'd be happy to be treated in their hospital. It was part of their public relations propaganda. After they found that just one in four members of staff would recommend the hospital where they worked to relatives or friends, or be happy to use it themselves, the question was quietly dropped. Would you take your car to a garage knowing that three out of four mechanics who worked there wouldn't trust the garage with their own car?) A third of Britain's general practitioners (GPs) would prefer private treatment for themselves and their families. Hospital consultants are the same. Here's what one NHS consultant had to say recently: `In the past we knew we would get good care on the NHS. I don't trust it any more. Even I can't bully my way through the system.' An increasing number of hospital doctors now buy private health care insurance so that they and their families won't have to endure NHS care. Trades unions defend the NHS and oppose any reforms but many of them have done deals with private sector organisations to provide private health care insurance so that their members don't have to use the NHS. More than half of the TUC's members have some sort of private medical insurance. This is a higher proportion than any other socio-economic group in the UK.

These people are all being wise. Tables which rank British hospitals invariably show that independent hospitals do much better than NHS hospitals in every measurable respect. Patients are treated better and they get better quicker. It is, perhaps, hardly surprising that just about every patient in the country (and every sane one) would, if given a choice, choose to have an operation in a private hospital rather than an NHS hospital. Politicians claim that they think the NHS is wonderful. They say that they wouldn't dream of going into a private hospital. But they don't have to wait to see a doctor and if they need in-patient treatment they go into private rooms where they are waited on hand and foot. They get private care without it costing them a penny.

The fact that the NHS is subject to endless lists of measured targets, productivity and incentives, is mainly due to the Labour Governments which began in 1997. Eventually, in November 2010, leading members of the medical establishment finally complained that the Government's target figures for hospital patients were affecting the quality of care provided. I had been criticising the provision of targets for at least a decade and it was always obvious that they were inappropriate for the provision of health care. The medical establishment does not, however, move quickly when it is faced the awful consequences of having to criticise any aspect of the NHS.

Hospitals are obsessed with curing (which they aren't terribly good at) and don't understand, or have time for, the principles of caring. For example, many hospitals refuse to allow visitors to take flowers into hospitals - arguing that flowers are a nuisance. This is sad. It has been known for thousands of years that patients are far more likely to get better quickly in hospitals which are bright, light, airy and filled with gentle music and fresh flowers. Since the first hospitals were built it has been recognised that the colour and perfume which flowers add to hospitals contribute greatly to the rate at which patients recover. Good hospitals are peaceful and are designed around a courtyard so that convalescent patients can walk in the cloisters and look at the flowers. But modern hospitals are designed for the convenience of the administrators. Patients are a bloody nuisance. I have recently been in several hospitals where the floors were carpeted because this made it nicer for the administrators when they were going to meetings. Naturally, the floors were stained with blood, urine and all the other remnants which would normally be wiped up off the floor. You can't ever properly clean a carpeted floor in a busy hospital because if the corridor is closed for proper cleaning the wards will be cut off. I know hospitals where the car park nearest the hospital entrance is reserved for administrators. Patients - however sick or frail they may be - have to walk, shuffle or limp half a mile in the rain. And why do hospitals clamp the cars of patients and visitors? Do they really think people want to spend more time than necessary in these places? Time and time again I have received letters from readers telling me that while having tests (and waiting to be seen at yet another department) they had, on top of all their other worries, been frightened that they would outstay the maximum three hour waiting period and would return to their vehicle to find it clamped.

I know of a hospital where the architect and bureaucrats put the psychiatric ward on the 6th floor. The ward had fully opening windows and a concrete walkway underneath. To everyone's astonishment the ward has a much higher rate of successful suicides than other comparable hospital psychiatric wards. The incidence of attempted suicides was no higher. But, despite a good many meetings, the administrators couldn't work out why the success rate among suicides was so high.

The vast majority of patients hand over their health (and their lives) to their doctors - without ever questioning what is happening to them. That is a dangerous way to live. Patients who take an interest in their own health may sometimes feel that the doctors and nurses who are looking after them regard them as a nuisance. But all the evidence shows clearly that such patients get better quicker, suffer fewer unpleasant side effects and live longer than patients who simply lie back passively and allow the professionals to take over. If your doctor wants you to take a drug make sure you know what to expect. If your doctor wants you to have surgery then make sure that you know what the surgery entails, what the possible consequences might be and what the alternatives are. Good questions to ask are: `Would you have this operation if you were me?' or: `Would you recommend this operation to someone in your close family?'

Hospitals are so bad that it is, perhaps, hardly surprising that I have for some years now recommended that every patient going into hospital should take a supply of disinfectant wipes, a mobile telephone, the telephone number of a local 24 hour taxi service and the phone numbers of at least three newspapers.

Remember: GPs kill retail but hospitals kill wholesale.

7. Doctors Are More Ignorant Than You (Or They) Think They Are.

When a doctor sees a patient he should, I believe, regard that patient as a member of his family. He should offer each patient the same level of treatment that he would offer his loved ones. Sadly, this does not happen these days. Many doctors now look at patients and wonder how quickly they can get rid of them - or how they can make the most money out of them. Doctors now frequently prescribe unnecessary drugs and perform unnecessary surgery. Today's doctors overprescribe, over-investigate and over-treat. They don't listen, they don't understand and they don't seem to care.

It isn't just GPs who are at fault, of course. According to a former Director General of the World Health Organisation: `The major and most expensive part of medical knowledge as applied today appears to be more for the satisfaction of the health profession than for the benefit of the consumers of health care.'

Animals receive better treatment than human patients. If you call for a vet you'll get one; call for a GP and you won't even be able to reach one, let alone speak to one. If your animal has a blood test you'll get the results back within minutes. If you have a blood test you'll be lucky to get the results in days and could end up waiting weeks. When our cat Thomasina needed a complex series of blood tests the vet visited our home and took the necessary blood samples.

She rang me back with the results about 15 minutes later. The fee for all this was, in medical terms, derisory.

Why the big difference? Vets provide a fee paid service without the State interfering. GPs work for the State and are paid, indirectly, via the general taxation system. Vets make home visits at day or night (and at reasonable costs) because they rely directly upon the customers for their income. GPs are now well paid, they work very few hours, they have long holidays, they do their very best to avoid home visits or night calls and they pass their difficult problems onto hospital specialists. A growing number of people are beginning to ask what GPs are for, and what they do to improve people's lives that could not be done by a prescription dispensing machine fitted, like a cash machine, into a convenient wall.

We are treated like children by doctors and told that we should allow them to make all the decisions. But the principles of health care (in all its aspects) are not difficult to understand and the people who pretend to be making the decisions for us don't know the truth because they have accepted what they have been told and have made no effort to look at the facts or request any evidence. To put it bluntly, they have been bought. The vast majority of doctors are whores.

Back in the early 1980s, I retired early from general practice to become a professional author. I took my name off the General Medical Council's register of practising doctors. I was suffering from chronic disillusionment. I was saddened and outraged by the way that the medical establishment had allowed itself to be controlled by the pharmaceutical industry and by the way the conspiracy between the two was ignoring the real needs of patients and needlessly damaging the health of hundreds of thousands of patients by encouraging the overuse of dangerous and sometimes lethal drugs. And I was appalled by the way that the deadening, cold fingers of medical bureaucracy were creeping into every aspect of medical practice and destroying the traditional, and in my eyes fundamental, relationship between the doctor and his patients.

I decided that I could do more good working outside the system. I hung up my stethoscope and permanently installed my typewriter on my desk.

I didn't intend to practise again and didn't imagine that I would ever again find myself needing to write out a prescription. Never say never. I recently put my name back on the General Medical Council's (GMC's) register of practising doctors. Go to the GMC website, key in my name and you will see that I am once again legally entitled to start a practice as a GP, get a hospital job or, indeed, open my own private hospital and offer heart surgery at Ł20,000 a pop or breast enlargement surgery for Ł1,000 an inch. It is not, however, my intention to do any of those things. I've gone back on the register not because I intend to start working as a GP again, or because I fancy getting a job in a hospital (who would), but simply so that I can, in an emergency, write out a prescription for an antibiotic or some other emergency essential. That's how bad I think it's become.

Thanks to a lethal mixture of lawyers, bureaucrats and politicians Britain's out of hours medical service is now virtually non-existent. A service which was for decades the envy of the world is now no more. It's deteriorating almost daily. One in five GP practices could soon close under Government proposals for super surgeries or polyclinics which will house up to 25 GPs and provide on-site pharmacies and a variety of other therapists. These are, of course, an EU 'proposal' and so despite the fact that neither doctors nor patients want them, the polyclinics will come. Polyclinics are much loved by socialists and have long flourished in communist eastern Europe.

A friend who visited his local GP yesterday told me that the receptionists at his doctor's surgery are now operating a triage system. The receptionists decide the order in which patients are seen according to their view on the seriousness of each patient's condition. Triage, the assessment of illnesses to decide the order of treatment of patients, used to be done by doctors. It's a business requiring much medical knowledge and the ability to make decisions quickly and accurately. Then, nurses started operating triage systems in hospital casualty departments. This was the first step in the dumbing down process. Now, with receptionists making clinical decisions, the system has reached rock bottom. How long will it be before receptionists are allowed to write prescriptions and stitch up the wounded?

Even practising doctors now recognise that there are huge problems with general practice. In March 2011, according to research conducted by *British Medical Journal Quality and Safety*, one in five British GPs admitted to having at least one incompetent colleague. This doesn't mean that one in five GPs has one colleague whom they didn't like or agree with. It means that one in five GPs regards at least one of their colleagues as *incompetent.*

Many of the doctors who had colleagues whom they regarded as incompetent admitted they did not report their views about their colleague to anyone in authority - partly for fear of retribution and partly because they suspected that nothing would happen.

And if one in five GPs is prepared to admit that he or she has incompetent colleagues how many GPs silently believe that they have incompetent colleagues? One in three? One in two? All of them?

A fellow with whom I was at medical school rang me up and asked me to go and visit him in his wonderful new health centre.

`You're a pretty forceful critic of modern medicine,' my acquaintance told me, although in truth I knew this already. I'll call him Keith, because that isn't his name. `You should come along and take a look around the new `state of the art' place we've had built.'

Always anxious to keep up with what is going on in the world of medicine I readily accepted his invitation.

And so I found myself tottering through huge plate glass doors and into a magnificent, purpose-built medical centre. White walls, white floor, white ceiling. A team of immaculately coiffed but fierce looking receptionists, all wearing spotless white coats, stood waiting behind bullet-proof, axe-proof glass partitions. Everywhere I looked there were signs telling me to do things or not to do things. There were more signs, warnings and threats than there are on the whole of the M25. I had to pinch myself to make sure that I hadn't died and gone to hell. I wasn't there because I was ill but the whole place reeked of sickness and death and made me feel queasy.

It all seemed such a very long way from the simple and rather homely surgeries in which medicine used to be practised. I remembered one very dear, former friend who practised in a tiny and rather cold conservatory built onto the side of his house. Patients sat waiting in his dining room where tattered, well-thumbed, old copies of *Country Life, Reader's Digest, Punch* and the *Dandy,* laid out on the dining table, provided the entertainment. The entertainment was needed for patients might have to wait some time to be seen. From time to time the doctor's stern and stout wife would potter into the room to check that no one was smoking, spitting or talking and to tidy the magazines up into neat piles. When my dear old chum was ready for his next patient he would shout `Next!' It was a simple technique but it worked and there was no reliance on wiring, electricity or other fallible consequences of the 20th century. When a consultation was over the patient, probably still buttoning up her dress or his trousers, would leave through the conservatory door, along the garden path and out through the side gate. This rather efficient system meant that there was never any congestion at the key point: the door between the dining room and the conservatory. Patients would happily queue for hours to see that doctor because he was kind and he understood and he cared. He was also the best diagnostician I've ever known. He couldn't read an X-ray and if you handed him a haematology report he'd be as flummoxed as if you'd given him the plans for a lunar rocketship but he had an instinct for sniffing out disease. And he knew his patients (most of whom he had brought into the world) so he knew when things were really wrong.

Keith proudly escorted me around the new building. There were, he explained, surgeries and examination rooms for the doctors, consulting rooms for the nurses and a small but well-equipped operating theatre for minor surgery. None of the doctors had their own room, of course. They just worked wherever the chief receptionist put them. This wasn't a place where you would find a picture of the doctor's family on his desk or a painting on a wall.

Keith seemed particularly proud of the pharmacy. And it was, I admit, an extremely impressive and extraordinarily well-stocked drug shop. It was the centre point of the whole building; a sort of pharmaceutical shrine at which all were expected to worship.

`Patients are processed in three simple stages,' he explained, rather in the manner of a tour guide taking visitors round a stately home. `First they are seen by the one of receptionists, who gives them a consultation number. Second, one of the doctors sees them. And then, finally, they visit the pharmacy to collect their prescription which will have been automatically ordered when the doctor completed his computerised record of the consultation. When collecting the prescription the patient is automatically given the date and time of their next appointment.'

`What about patients who don't need a prescription?' I asked.

The fellow with whom I had been at medical school stared at me. `What do you mean?' he asked, genuinely puzzled.

I tried to redesign the question. `What happens to patients who need another appointment but don't need treatment with drugs?'

Keith stared at me. `All patients need treatment,' he said. `Why else would someone visit us if they didn't need treatment?'

`Well, I think the idea that all patients need treatment is arguable,' I said, feeling rather like the small boy declaring that the Emperor was wearing no clothes. `But what about those patients who need treatment but don't need drugs?'

`How else would we treat them?' asked the doctor, clearly puzzled.

'I don't know,' I shrugged. 'It rather depends on what is wrong with them. Osteopathy, acupuncture, dietary advice, relaxation exercises, meditation training...'

I stopped talking because I was aware that my former colleague was looking rather alarmed.

'I hadn't realised that you were one of those nutters,' he said, pulling his white coat around him, as though it were a suit of armour which would protect him from contamination. He instinctively backed away a few inches.

'Surely some patients might just need someone to talk to?' I suggested, rather lamely.

'It's obviously been a little while since you practised,' said my former colleague, rather coldly.

I left there feeling rather sad and even depressed; convinced, more than ever, that medicine has been taken over by the hugely powerful and immensely profitable pharmaceutical industries.

Doctors are no longer in the business of caring for patients. They are in the much simpler business of dishing out pills. This is partly the fault of doctors and the medical profession. But it is, ultimately, the responsibility of politicians who have, once again, failed the people they were elected to serve.

The Government (with the aid and support of the bureaucrats in Brussels and the tacit approval of the medical establishment) seems determined to destroy general practice. Whether this is a deliberate policy or a consequence of egregious incompetence only they can possibly know.

Bureaucrats who negotiated the deal allowing GPs to avoid 24 hour responsibility showed just how poorly they understood the basic principle of GP care.

GPs were offered the chance to hand over all their out of hours work to agencies because of EU laws limiting their working hours. The European Working Time Directive limits the working time for everyone - including doctors - to 48 hours a week. There is no room for flexibility and so doctors either have to abandon patients half way through emergency treatment, if their time is up, or they have to lie on their time sheets. Otherwise, there's a big fine to pay the EU. (The fact that doctors are now filling in time sheets is reason enough to leave the EU. The fact that the EU fines our hospitals for not obeying its rules is another reason.) All this is bad enough in hospital where, in the bad old days, junior doctors worked in teams with senior doctors and could, and did, follow patients through from admittance to discharge. But now doctors float around, making sure that there are doctors somewhere in the hospital. Doctors don't see patients through from start to finish and have no idea whether treatments worked or failed or made the patient worse. And, naturally, patients get no continuity. But this new legislation has destroyed general practice. The whole traditional basis of general practice is that the family doctor takes full 365 day a year responsibility for his patients. Without that role GPs have no purpose and could best be replaced by a combination of walk-in clinics (staffed 24 hours a day) and an enhanced ambulance service. Now that GPs don't work 'out of hours' (presumably because bureaucrats believe that illness only strikes in normal office hours), administrators have to take responsibility for providing some sort of cover so that patients who are inconsiderate enough to fall ill or have accidents at weekends, evenings and nights can be dealt with.

Over the Christmas holidays a friend spent two desperate days trying to find a doctor prepared to see his wife (who was suffering from a sudden and troublesome infection and who clearly urgently needed antibiotics). He eventually managed to speak to a doctor on the telephone. But the doctor couldn't visit, or see patients, because he was providing medical cover for heaven knows how many patients, spread over several hundred square miles of England. The condition had to wait until after the holidays - by which time, of course, it had deteriorated considerably.

Other friends and readers have told me similar stories. At night and at weekends it is virtually impossible to see a doctor. If you try really hard you can get to talk to one on the phone. But that's it. Outside London there are very few private general practitioners and most GPs now work shorter hours than people who work for the local council. (Compared to their predecessors they also look after surprisingly few patients. List sizes have shrunk to a fraction of what they were.)

It is because it is now almost impossible to find weekend medical treatment that I went back onto the medical register. I don't have any patients but I want to be able to have access to life-saving drugs in case I or my wife need emergency medical help.

Doctors in general practice leapt at the chance to work civil service hours because most of them are utterly disillusioned and fed-up. A generation ago doctors went into general practice with a sense of honest purpose and public service. Today it's just about the money. The problem with doctors today is not that they are stupid (you don't actually need much intelligence to be a doctor) but that they lack imagination, common sense, empathy, humanity and passion. And they have no sense of commitment and service. Today's doctors have no vocation and no sense of responsibility to the community they serve. You can teach the science of medicine but you can't teach the art, the instinct, the passion or the dedication. A medical student who does not start his working life with these qualities is unlikely to pick them up on the way. And yet instinct and imagination are vital skills for a doctor who wishes to excel as a diagnostician.

Now that GPs are working 30 to 40 hour weeks the authorities are having to struggle hard to find doctors prepared to work as locums and to cover the out of hours work. And since there aren't enough qualified British GPs prepared to do this work the authorities have to import doctors from other European countries. The EU rules allow a doctor from one EU country to work in any other European country, regardless of whether or not he speaks that country's language. (So, for example, because I am qualified and registered and licensed as a British doctor I am entitled to practise in Italy or

Greece despite the fact that I do not speak a word of Italian or Greek.)

There are many ways in which Government run, State sponsored health care does genuine harm. So, for example, the Government `encourages' general practitioners to run appointment systems even though there is little doubt that both patients and doctors are better off without them. When I first practised as a GP in the early 1970s I had no appointment system. Patients turned up at my surgery, sat in the waiting room and waited. If there was a long queue they would pop out, do some shopping, and come back half an hour later. The system worked well. I don't remember anyone ever complaining. I employed one receptionist to take the patients' names and make sure that I was supplied with the appropriate medical records.

And then the bureaucrats decided that I had to organise an appointment system. Patients had to ring up in advance to make a date to see me. Teams of receptionists had to be employed to take messages and keep the appointment book. Emergencies still had to be slotted in. The whole system was a disaster. I sometimes found that patients were having to wait several days to see me. Patients complained that the telephone line was engaged. Cancellations resulted in the appointment book becoming incomprehensible. Patients who had to wait 15 minutes (because I was running late) complained.

I still usually held `open' surgeries on bank holidays and at weekends. Patients would turn up, sit in the waiting room and be seen in turn. Just like the `bad' old days. No one complained. There were no arguments. Everyone knew who was next in line. And the system worked efficiently and well.

Appointment systems were introduced to please bureaucrats and to provide employment for masses of low-grade clerks. The bureaucrats who run the NHS couldn't bear the idea of any aspect of the health service being run without a need for vast numbers of clerks and administrators. Today, appointment systems have become a major problem and should be scrapped. The clerks who make the appointments have grabbed as much power as they possibly can and have risen far above themselves. Health centre deceptionists talk glibly about how they use a `triage' system to arrange appointments. Some use the word as though they know what it means. These clerks know nothing about medicine but somehow assume that they are able to make decisions about whether or not patient A is more needy than patient B.

Patients, quite rightly do not like appointment systems and nor do doctors who care about what patients like. (Some greedy GPs have so much contempt for their patients that - until they were banned - they introduced premium rate telephone lines so that patients ringing to make appointments had to pay huge fees for the privilege of doing so.)

I strongly suspect that any private GP who set up a practice without an appointment system would attract more patients than he could cope with. If, in addition, he provided an out of hours service (for a fee, of course) he would become the most popular GP in the country. The problem, of course, is that most doctors wouldn't have the foggiest how to run a private practice, and they know it. They have grown rich and lazy working in the NHS.

But the bureaucrats are determined to keep appointments. Indeed, things are going to get much, much worse. There are plans to introduce a national appointment service. Patients will ring a single telephone number and (if they get through before they die) they will speak to a faceless, nameless operator (probably working in India) who will (if the computer is working) give them an appointment to suit the system. Centralised appointment booking will be introduced because it will be convenient and economical for the bureaucrats. Patients will lose out. But no one cares about them.

Patients would overwhelmingly prefer to go back to the days when they could just turn up at their local surgery and see the doctor of their choice simply by sitting and waiting for a few minutes or even an hour or so. For patients the old-fashioned way of doing things was cheaper and far more convenient. And it resulted in much faster treatment too.

Appointment systems aren't the only problem, of course.

When I was a GP I found that I was constantly having to find ways to defend my patients from the bureaucrats. Once, for example, a State bureaucrat arrived and announced that he was going to take away all the medical records I held for my 2,500 patients. He had a van parked outside my surgery, ready to take the records away with him. I pointed out that this would be a breach of confidentiality and would endanger the lives of my patients. The bureaucrat wouldn't budge. He had a form giving him the right to remove the records for routine checking. He asked me to take a medical record file from its drawer and to read what was written in red on the bottom of the file. I did so. It said: `The property of the Minister of Health'. Suddenly I remembered Shylock and the *Merchant of Venice*. `You can take the records,' I told him. `But you can't take the ink.' He stared at me, uncomprehendingly. `The paper belongs to the Minister of Health,' I conceded. `But the ink on the paper belongs to me. So you can take the records but you must leave the ink behind.'

He left. No one ever bothered me again.

Things today are rather different.

I received a letter from a reader in Scotland who advised me that he had been told by his doctor that before he could receive treatment he had to sign a `counter fraud declaration'. He wanted to know what it was. (His GP didn't seem to know or care.) I discovered that patients registering at practices in Scotland are required to sign one of these documents (containing sensitive, personal ID information) before they can receive any treatment. The declaration entitles the doctor to share the patient's information with a variety of Government agencies including the UK Border Agency, the Department for Work and Pensions and HM Revenue and Customs. In other words: everyone over the age of 16.

Doctors in Scotland moaned a bit about the blatant breach of confidentiality, but did nothing. Since the Government is the body wanting the information it's fair to assume that the GMC will have approved this outrageous abuse of patient confidentiality.

It is, perhaps, hardly surprising that most doctors now hate their jobs and regard them as little more than a way of making money. Many doctors would prefer to do something else for a living - if they could find something as lucrative. Vocation has been abandoned and replaced by expediency. Doctors and nurses who truly care simply leave or take retirement as soon as they can.

In what are now regarded as the 'bad old days' doctors had little else to offer but kindness and understanding and relied upon the placebo effect of their personalities. Patients often got better because they believed. Today, doctors think they are scientists and think they know everything. But they don't. And by ignoring the placebo response they miss out on 50% of their healing power. Doctors in the 'bad old days' needed to be charming in order to attract patients and to be paid. Doctors working for the State, or for insurance companies, don't have to worry about having a good bedside manner. It is, many seem to feel, beneath them.

In my view, things went wrong for doctors when they became civil servants. GPs should be self-employed and run their practices without interference. Traditionally, GPs have always been the backbone of any health care provisions - acting as guides and champions for patients struggling to use the system. But today's GPs do not run the system. There are two reasons for this. First, modern GPs have shown no backbone or moral fibre. They are concerned only with getting the best financial deal for themselves. Second, other NHS employers (nurses, social workers, administrators and, quite probably, hospital car park attendants) have been vocal and determined in their insistence that they should be treated as equals within the NHS system. The result: chaos.

British GPs now earn more than ever, and do less useful work than ever. They are paid more, and have received higher pay rises in recent years, than their counterparts anywhere else in the world. Under recent Governments the income of British GPs has jumped sixfold. And yet during that same period the service provided has deteriorated at an extraordinary rate. GPs now spend much (sometimes most) of their reduced working week dealing with paperwork. None of this nonsense makes patients safer or healthier.

As a result of GPs cutting down their working hours, seriously ill patients may have to wait ten hours for a doctor to call. A few locum GPs (who don't know the patients they see, don't have access to their medical records and may or may not speak very much English) now race around providing emergency care in a bizarre and utterly inadequate way. One woman in South Wales who wanted a visit from a GP was told that the nearest doctor was in Sheffield. Another, living in the same part of the country, was told that the nearest available doctor was 300 miles away in Cleveland. The relatively small number of GPs hired to provide out of hours services are, inevitably, reluctant to visit anyone. Their area of responsibility extends so far that some seem to prefer to deal with emergencies on the telephone. I have, in the past, failed in my attempts to obtain emergency medical treatment for friends and relatives. The inevitable result is that most people simply ring for an ambulance - putting enormous, additional and unnecessary strain on the ambulance service and on overstretched Accident and Emergency services.

Astonishingly, GPs now want to cut down home and surgery visits still further. The plan is for GPs to offer e-mail diagnoses. Patients will e-mail their symptoms and the GP will say whether they need to visit the surgery. This is possibly one of the most arrogant, stupid, selfish, unprofessional and dangerous ideas I have ever heard of. It will result in the incidence of doctor-induced disease becoming commoner than heart disease, stroke and cancer combined. I have for years refused to offer advice by mail to my readers on the grounds that it simply isn't safe for any doctor to do so. It's not surprising that many patients now choose to see alternative practitioners who may, or may not, be qualified and competent. Many simply seek advice from an assistant in their local health food store.

The ways in which the politicians and the bureaucrats interfere seem to grow almost weekly. Doctors are now bribed by the Government to increase the number of times they diagnose certain diseases. So, for example, GPs receive a cash bonus if they manage to diagnose a certain number of patients as suffering from Chronic Obstructive Pulmonary Disease (COPD). These patients will then usually be given prescription drugs for the rest of their lives. It doesn't take the brain of an Einstein to work out who benefits from this scheme. Once patients have been labelled the drug company profits will soar. And the incidence of doctor (and drug) induced disease will also soar.

Most GPs make little or no attempt to teach their patients anything, or to look out for early signs or symptoms of disease. When check-ups are performed they are done, by rote, by nurses who simply follow a pre-determined pattern of questions and advice and who, by and large, know something between very little and nothing useful about medicine. GPs rarely bother to organise routine checks on elderly patients (who might benefit) because there are no bonus payments for doing these.

The average GP now works a four day week. She has nights and weekends off. She is available on the telephone one day a week. She does home visits one day a week. She is paid according to `performance related activities'. Practices are driven to satisfy targets (so many patients vaccinated, so many treated for heart disease and so on). As a result, the average GP no longer provides any sort of personal service. She spends 15 hours a week with patients and is paid around Ł120,000 a year. Family doctors are now doing less work for more money. Many GPs now earn Ł250,000 a year or more for working hours that would not alarm a librarian. Today's primary care service is run by and for bureaucrats. Doctors can no longer choose where they work. And patients can no longer choose the doctor they want to see. Modern doctors are controlled by bureaucrats and so they themselves think and behave like bureaucrats. What a tragedy.

As they've become richer so GPs have become less competent - and constantly ready to adopt ways of working which diminish their likelihood of providing their patients with a good service. The interview is the most important part of the doctors diagnostic equipment. That's when he talks to the patient and - even more important than talking, though you wouldn't think so if you sit in on the average clinic - listens to what the patient has to say. It is by listening to patients that doctors learn most. But over the years doctors have accumulated more and more equipment to help them make diagnoses. Too often the doctor relies exclusively on his equipment; trusting it implicitly to provide him with the right answers. The more complex modern medical equipment has become the worse medical treatment has become.

The first piece of equipment that doctors acquired was the stethoscope. This now symbolic device was invented so that doctors could listen to their patients' chests without having to put their heads down on their bosoms. The stethoscope added to the doctor's dignity. But it also provided the first mechanical barrier between doctor and patient. And since René Laennec first introduced the stethoscope the doctor patient relationship has been weakened and damaged by this obsession with equipment. A few years ago a study at Harvard University showed that many patients who had died would have still been alive if the doctors looking after them had relied upon their heads instead of equipment that was often poorly set up or badly calibrated. (Hospital doctors are just as bad at understanding the equipment they use. It is not uncommon for sales representatives to be present in operating theatres when equipment they have supplied is being used. They are there not just to give advice but to provide practical help. There are many people around who have been operated on not by surgeons but by sales representatives. I doubt if anyone knows how many patients the sales representatives have killed.

Diagnosis should be better these days. But it is often much worse. When I was a young doctor (back in the 1970s) the older doctors all relied on their intuition and their `feel' for patients. I knew doctors who could make accurate diagnoses time and time again. And when they did not know what was wrong they knew that something was wrong. Today, doctors rely on tests and machinery and they make far more mistakes than before.

Medicine has become a `business' rather than a profession - if you have any doubts about that just look at the number of doctors who now go on strike, or threaten to go on strike, in order to improve their personal pay. Like all businessmen, modern doctors are influenced by profit rather than any other motive when considering what to do. A continuing association with a ruthless industry which constantly favours profit at the expense of everything else has rubbed off on the profession. When the British Medical Association (BMA) talked about industrial action in June 2011 it was to protest about the Government's sensible plan to revise GPs pensions. (Before threatening a strike, the BMA should have studied history. As I have pointed out, mortality rates invariably fall when doctors go on strike.)

In addition to having a responsibility to their own patients, doctors have responsibilities to patients in general, to themselves as physicians and to their profession. Sadly, most have abandoned all of those responsibilities. Doctors fail to protect the public against polluted drinking water and food packed with carcinogens. GPs don't stand up and make their collective voice heard about these important issues because their interests are now allied too closely with those of the drug companies and the State. And so doctors support vaccination (a dangerous and unproven practice) because the system has made it profitable for them. In my first book *The Medicine Men* (published in 1975), I wrote that doctors who take orders from a trade can hardly describe themselves as belonging to a profession. I was pilloried for that. But it's truer now than it was then.

Doctors who have kept quiet about changes which have resulted in appallingly inadequate services for patients, must share collective guilt for the storm of unnecessary deaths and the injuries caused by the profession as a whole. Medical deaths and injuries are now endemic.

Modern doctors think that medicine is a science. It isn't. The new doctors miss the diagnostic nuances which are essential because they simply don't see medicine as an art or a craft; they live by mechanical, diagnostic rules. It is diagnosis by rote. Treating people by numbers. It is not surprising that many actually believe that computers could do the job just as well. The new doctors prefer to rely on laboratory results. Ambitious, young doctors qualify and move up the ladder with frighteningly little practical experience.

The result is that when a doctor sees a patient with an unusual symptom, or a symptom which doesn't quite fit with his computer-like expectations, he is inclined to dismiss it or ignore it. He doesn't realise that all patients are different and that not all patients fit what the books say. Doctors tend to depend entirely upon laboratory tests rather than clinical experience or wisdom and they don't realise that tests can be, and often are, terrifyingly misleading. The result is that there is not much original or creative thinking in medicine. The art is being driven out of the profession. All this helps explain why doctors now make so many terrible mistakes. (Doctors tend to rely on tests because paperwork can be produced in court as evidence for making a diagnosis. Doctors who rely on intuition have more difficulty in explaining the reasons for their diagnosis. Litigious patients and greedy lawyers are partly responsible for the dangerous deterioration in the quality of medical practice.)

Today's doctors are too important (and too reliant on their equipment) to see patients in their own homes. What a huge mistake that is. The doctor who sees his patients in their homes will understand them, their families, their health, their susceptibility to illness far more than the doctor who spends her or his working lifetime sitting behind a desk. Incidentally, it isn't only GPs who don't often see patients in their own homes. Hospital consultants don't see patients at home much, either. Just a few years ago hospital consultants often saw patients at home. And I suspect that even fewer GPs now visit their patients in hospital to make sure that they are being well looked after - and that they understand what is happening to them. When I was a GP, just a few decades ago, I regularly visited my patients in hospital. And I regularly arranged for specialists to visit them at home.

Modern doctors get things wrong because they don't usually go back to sources. They rely on what they have been told by drug company representatives, Government employed bureaucrats and politicians - all of whom have a vested interest in putting forward a particular line and none of whom are likely to know the truth or where to find it (or even what it looks like).

Doctors may, of course, think they can rely on medical journals and published research work. They may read books, magazines or newsletters which rely on material extracted from journal articles. But they won't get the truth there either I'm afraid. Some of the frequently quoted medical journals accept research articles for money. The vast majority of papers published in medical and scientific journals are of little or no value; indeed, many are fraudulent and misleading. The paper which looks as if it is independent may have been published because some corporation (usually a drug company) has paid for it to be published. Nearly all journals accept and rely on advertising (and it is difficult to remain open-minded when you will go bankrupt if you do). And finally most of the scientists who write journal articles have a vested interest in the product or treatment they are writing about. Many receive grants or payments for the work they do, or they own shares in the company making the product they are (allegedly) researching. Scientific papers are rarely exactly what they seem to be and though they may be quoted and used as references there is a real danger that they may be worse than useless. Drug companies control what is published by limiting the publication of critical research. In order to read scientific papers successfully it is necessary to know how to interpret what you find (and how to read between the lines). Since much medical education is dominated by the pharmaceutical industry students are not taught how to do this. It would be inconvenient if too many people knew just how easy it is to manipulate medical research to fit commercial needs.

I've been digging out the truth for nearly 40 years and I have made a lot of enemies in doing it. I know all the tricks the drug companies and food companies use. Researchers know that to please their masters they must simply ask the question which is most likely to give them the answer they want. Financially inconvenient results are ignored or shelved or overlooked.

Because of the books I've written on medicine, I regularly hear medical horror stories. For example, a reader of mine had a pain in her leg. She rang her doctor at about 8.00 p.m. The doctor who made the diagnosis (on the telephone, of course) told my reader that she had a deep vein thrombosis and should stay flat on her back in bed and do nothing until the next morning when she should take himself along to the local hospital. The doctor, from an agency of some kind, did not explain how my reader, who lives alone and has no car, should make the journey from bedroom to hospital.

It's hardly surprising that an increasing number of people die unnecessarily. It's hardly surprising that the number of complaints made against doctors increases annually.

Most doctors kill through incompetence and carelessness rather than through design and malice. But the end result is the same.

Many illness can be easily prevented. But the problem is that if doctors take the steps which will prevent those illnesses they will annoy big businesses. And doctors don't like putting themselves at risk these days. So doctors continue to ask the wrong questions and do the wrong things. And patients are beginning to notice that the big differences in the quality of care provided are dependent not so much upon the area of the country they live in but the enthusiasm and decency of the doctor to whom they have been allotted (but whom they may, in practice, see only rarely). The official figures are simply awful. There is an eightfold variation in the rate at which patients with suspected cancer are referred to specialists. A third of patients with stomach and throat cancers are given non-urgent referrals when they should have been regarded as urgent. There are also massive but entirely unjustified variations in prescribing practices. It is impossible to guess just how many people are killed each year by incompetent GPs but there is absolutely no doubt that, as I said, in my book *How To Stop Your Doctor Killing You*: `The person most likely to kill you is not a burglar, a mugger, a deranged relative or a drunken driver. The person most likely to kill you is your doctor.'

The bottom line is that doctors should work for patients and no one else. (They have wider responsibilities to the community but their primary responsibility is to their patients.) State and insurance health schemes have destroyed this relationship by allowing or encouraging doctors to see things a different way. The modern doctor is employed by the State or insurance company and has come to regard her employer as the primary object of her loyalty.

When I was younger I thought it was just the drug companies which were corrupt. Now I realise that masses of people in the medical establishment are corrupt. I suspect that each group thinks that their profession is the only one run by bad people but I fear the sad truth is that every establishment group is run by bad people for bad reasons.

Today, you can't believe much that doctors tell you. The reason? They themselves know far less than you (and they) think they know. Doctors rarely know the truth about anything. They are lied to by their employers and by the drug companies. Many of the journals they read are paid for or subsidised by the advertising they contain.

Most of us choose our barber or our car mechanic with great care. We look around, we ask people we know and trust, we make judgements based on our past experience. But we don't choose doctors in the same way. We take what we get and assume that they are trustworthy. We are told by the bureaucrats which family doctor we can see and must then hope that we haven't been allocated to a doctor who is depressed, psychotic, uncaring or egregiously incompetent.

I suspect that people who aren't angry about what has happened to health care in Britain still don't understand just how bad things have become; how corrupt and venal doctors have become. I have this recurrent nightmare. I telephone for a doctor. It is night-time. It is an emergency. The telephone is answered by a machine. A voice speaks. Press 1 if you are dying and require an undertaker. Press 2 if you are dying and wish to donate organs before seeing an undertaker.

I wake in a sweat and wonder how long it will be before my nightmare becomes a bureaucrat's daydream.

8. Cowgirl Nurses With Great Expectations

Traditionally, nurses are beyond criticism. They are `angels' and they have always received a `good press'. But nurses have changed. And they have changed a good deal. The result is that today's nurses are nothing like their predecessors. If they are to be forced back into doing what they should be doing then they need to be criticised - and their shortcomings need to be identified.

The big problem is that today's nurses are too self-important to carry out any of the traditional tasks entrusted to nurses. Modern nurses don't like to bother much with caring, touching, feeding or comforting. They regard themselves as above collecting bedpans or plumping up pillows. Nurses are now too self-important to feed patients or to lift them and too protective of their past to let anyone else do these things either. It is a tragedy that as nurses have become too important to nurse, no other group has been allowed to take on the most essential caring tasks. Auxiliaries, for example, are not allowed to do anything with to or for patients and the result is that there is no one on the average hospital ward to wash, feed or care for patients.

In the bad old days nurses would help their patients in a thousand tiny ways. They would make sure that their female patients wore clean nighties and had their hair brushed before visiting time. They don't do these things any more. And it isn't that they have other, more important things to do. Go into any hospital these days and you will see half a dozen nurses sitting around the nurses' station chatting and eating chocolates. (It's no wonder they're all so fat. You'd think nurses would be more concerned with their health. If they got up and moved about a bit occasionally they would burn up some of the calories.)

Nurses should bandage wounds, make beds, empty bedpans and soothe sweaty brows. They should take temperatures and record pulse rates and give out prescribed medicines. That's what they are there for and it's what they are best at. It is also what patients need from them. These are important tasks. Sadly, most nurses consider themselves far too grand for such work. Nurses have become lazy. It is their responsibility to make sure that hospitals are kept spotlessly clean and that patients with dangerous infections are barrier nursed. But nurses consider themselves too important to deal with practical issues. They prefer to sit around having meetings with social workers. On many wards these days it is impossible to find a nurse. Patients who need one must wait until one appears and then try to catch her attention. Sympathy and comfort are not qualities required of nurses these days. Indeed, I suspect that they are regarded as unsuitable weaknesses. Today's Mrs Gamp is too busy attending meetings to attend her patients. Mrs Gamp has acquired ideas well above her station.

In some hospitals these days the sheets aren't changed when patients leave and patients arrive. Instead, to save money, the sheets are just turned over. Top to bottom. The sort of practice that is frowned upon in the sleaziest of seaside boarding houses. It is, of course, the administrators who decide that this will be done. But it is the nurses who supervise its doing. (It's the auxiliaries who do the actual work, of course. Nurses don't do physical stuff any more.) And so the nurses are responsible. Just as they are responsible for allowing men and women to be put onto the same ward, and forced to share the same bathrooms and lavatories. Why don't nurses stand up against these despicable practices? Easy. They say nothing because they have been institutionalised. They work for the Government and they don't have the guts or the intelligence to realise that if they say 'no' the authorities won't dare do anything to them.

Many of today's nurses are graduates; awash with diplomas and certificates. But their patients lie in their own faeces and urine. They do not have their faces washed or their teeth brushed or their nails cut or their hair combed. These are things that are beneath the new graduate nurse. Today's graduate nurses are too busy chatting and playing with their computers to check that there is soap in the bathroom or toilet paper in the lavatory. Graduate nurses are different from their predecessors in that they are never around when needed. They tut and look cross if they are disturbed and asked to do something practical. Nurses, like administrators, have acquired authority but shed responsibility. There is no sense of caring. There is no accountability, no discipline and no supervision. When things go wrong (as they often do) no one is blamed except, possibly, the patients. Nurses chase promotion, attend seminars and perform useless research. They demand to be given time to attend to their office duties and to attend meetings. They insist on personal project time, time for research work and study time. There are, in short, many chiefs but no Indians. The young people who go into nursing with great aims and ideals are quickly broken and destroyed.

They still have a sort of ward sister in hospitals but these days she is far too important to do anything practical. These superior nurses, full of qualifications but empty of compassion, sit in cubbyholes, with the door closed. They share their cubbyholes with a computer screen, a packet of biscuits, many grievances and much ambition. They spend their days plotting how to gain more power from the administrators. (They've already beaten the doctors to a bloody pulp.)

Because nurses are now too important, and too busy with their administrative chores, to deal with patients, hospitals now employ untrained assistants to attend to patients. These assistants prepare patients for medical procedures. For example, my wife went to see a radiologist. The man who entered her cubicle, asked her to remove her clothing and then smeared petroleum jelly onto her abdomen was a young hospital employee who had no medical qualifications. He could have been working in the bank. Instead he was allowed to attend to female patients. By himself.

Modern nurses seem to be trying to reposition themselves as the new cheap doctors. They are managed to acquire for themselves the right to prescribe and to perform surgical procedures. (I am surprised incidentally that the British Medical Association, the doctors' trade union has not moaned about this. As nurses have acquired more of the powers traditionally reserved for doctors so an increasing number of young doctors have found themselves unemployed - forced to collect dole money or to leave the country to find employment.) Nurses are being given more power (and allowed to make diagnoses, prescribe drugs, perform surgery and make life or death decisions) because this is good for the State. Nurses are cheaper to train and less expensive to employ than doctors. However, allowing nurses to have these extra powers is exceedingly bad for patients because nurses are even more likely than doctors to make serious errors when attempting to treat patients.

The news that nurses are to be allowed to decide which patients should - or should not - be resuscitated is terrifying news that should frighten the life out of every patient, every relative and every potential patient - and that means all of us.

My main objection is that nurses simply don't have the training to make this sort of decision. Nurses should stick to making beds and reading thermometers and caring for patients and they should stop trying to turn themselves into fake doctors. The horrifying incidence of superbugs in British hospitals proves without a doubt that nurses aren't doing their present jobs properly. The nursing profession has gone rapidly down hill since nurses decided that simply `nursing' patients wasn't enough for them.

Another problem created by giving nurses extra responsibilities of this type is that the traditional relationship between nurse and patient has been changed dramatically - and for the worse. Nurses now either have to hold back from real contact with their patients (in which case they are failing them) or they have to get to know them (in the traditional, caring way) and then decide whether they live or die (in which case they will fail them because they won't be able to make the right decision).

Sadly, the modern nurse seems to be ashamed to be a nurse; she wants to be a clinical professional. She wants to perform procedures, prescribe drugs, operate computers and attend meetings. Lots of meetings. It is considered demeaning for a nurse to provide caring these days. They want to be doctors without the pain of a long, expensive education. Nurses want to grab the power the cheap and easy way, without having to spend six years at university. They want equality of money and power with doctors, without actually having to do all the hard work. And so the nursing profession has lost its way.

There is, of course, a simple solution to this dilemma. Nurses who want to pretend that they are doctors should train and become doctors. And that, of course, is the problem. The vast majority of nurses are, quite simply, incapable of completing a medical degree course. They are, to be blunt, not quite bright enough.

Things started to go wrong in the nursing profession when self-deluded, self-important nurses decided that they wanted to be treated as academics rather than as nurses. Nursing used to be a sacred vocation. Now it's just a career. I go into a lot of hospitals and the situation almost everywhere is the same. Bedbound patients desperately ring their bells needing attention while overweight nurses sit in meetings drinking coffee and eating biscuits. I have even been in hospitals where nurses regularly refuse to lift patients. `That's not what we're here for,' one told me. `We're not weightlifters.'

It's about time someone remembered that nursing is a crucial part of medical care. And nurses should be proud to be nurses.

If you want evidence supporting the low quality of nursing care just look at the hospital infection figures. Britain has the highest incidence of Methicillin Resistant Staphylococcus Aureus (MRSA) infection in the world. There's only one reason for that: sloppy nursing. Nurses don't wash their hands between patients. I've seen them go in and out of rooms where patients with MRSA were being nursed without washing or even wiping their hands. Garage mechanics have cleaner hands than most nurses.

Things have got so bad that the relatives of patients in hospital now need to take in antiseptic wipes and clean beds, tables and lockers every day because the staff won't do this. Patients need to have antiseptic wipes so that they can clean their cutlery.

And bedsores are now so common that no one notices them. Today's nurses just regard them as `normal'. With rare exceptions any patient who develops a bedsore has not been properly nursed. Bedsores used to be regarded as a sign of bad nursing. These days they are simply a sign that a patient has been in hospital for more than a couple of weeks.

Nursing ambition has been disastrous for patient care. Misled by the enthusiasms of the over-ambitious and the commercially-minded too much effort has gone into curing and too little into caring. Ironically, there is ample evidence hidden in the world's medical journals to show that a caring approach is not simply compassionate but is also effective. In a paper which appeared in the *New England Journal of Medicine* in America, doctors showed that when pregnant women are given the sort of support that can best be given by a kind nurse with a little time to spend, women delivered their babies in half the time and suffered far fewer complications. Many other papers have illustrated the same point: patients need less technology and more care.

Meanwhile, the present system ensures that the nurses who run hospitals, who make the rules and who provide the `leadership' are the ones who are least capable of, and least interested in, working directly with patients. The nurses who are in charge are the ones who are least interested in the art of caring, least passionate about nursing as an art and most anxious to climb up the career ladder by exhibiting their prowess at managing meetings, mastering the double-speak that has invaded hospitals and giving 'good mouth'. Nursing lost its way when it became impossible for a nurse to rise in the hierarchy without becoming an administrator. Nursing went wrong when nurses started collecting diplomas and degrees. How can you have a degree in caring?

A few decades ago patients were cared for in hospitals which were run by matrons and ward sisters - nurses who still knew how to turn a patient, make a bed and empty a bedpan. Most patients cannot, of course, remember how efficient hospitals were in those days and so, because they don't know what to expect or what to look for, think they are being well looked after. Most people have low expectations, are inherently grateful for anything that is done for them, are frightened and don't know what to look for. (This is the only possible explanation for those letters to local newspapers extolling the virtues of the local hospital.) These days the brigades of fat-bottomed nurses who `administer' our hospitals are too self-important even to look at patients, let alone speak to them. You can occasionally spot these nursing administrators darting along the corridors, eyes averted lest they accidentally soil their vision with the sight of someone in pyjamas or a nightdress. Most of the time these nursing harridans lie hidden behind office doors, planning their career progress. Many of them seem grossly obese - a consequence no doubt of doing too little work and spending too much time drinking coffee and munching biscuits. If the salaries of these grotesque beasts were smaller, and they spent less time in meetings, there would be plenty of time and money to make sure that agency nurses were unnecessary. (There is very little continuity in nursing care in modern hospitals. Patients are lucky if they ever see the same nurse twice.) Meanwhile, those nurses who are left at the dirty end of the profession, wander around almost uninterested in their work. Often slovenly and untidy, they do not seem to care for their patients at all. It is frequently difficult, if not impossible, to tell who is in charge. The modern nurses' office (or `station') will usually be positioned in a spot where the nurses can hide away from the patients to make their phone calls, eat their chocolates and gossip. Inevitably, if the patients cannot see the nurses, the converse is also true: the nurses cannot see the patients. Calls for help or bedpans go unnoticed.

Today's nurses are grotesquely unprofessional and are, far too often, rude to patients and visitors. I have received numerous complaints of hospital nurses talking loudly at night (and keeping patients awake). This is quite unnecessary. It is also rude and bad medicine. When I last worked in hospital, doctors and nurses would whisper even when working on emergencies so as not to waken patients. Today's nurses are badly trained. And most don't seem to know how a good hospital should be run.

Ever since the Greeks built the first hospitals it has been recognised that flowers are good for patients. They look good. They smell good. They bring the healing beauty of nature into the ward. But flowers are banned in many modern hospitals. They are considered to be a nuisance.

When I last took flowers to a patient in hospital the nurses looked at me as though I were a madman. After I pointed out that I had bought the flowers in the hospital shop one grudgingly agreed that the hospital didn't ban flowers. `I don't do flowers,' said the nurse, as indignantly as if I'd asked her to put on a nice little pinny and bake me a cake. So I found a cleaner. And asked her for help. `I don't do flowers,' said the cleaner, looking down her nose. Judging by the state of the ward she didn't do much cleaning either. Eventually, I found a vase in a filthy cupboard and filled it myself with water. I then put the flowers into the vase, arranged them and left them on the table by the bed. Half an hour after I left, the flowers were thrown out.

9. Medicine Is Not A Science

Orthodox medical practitioners like to give the impression that they have conquered sickness with science but there are, at a conservative estimate, something in the region of 18,000 known diseases for which there are still no effective treatments - let alone cures. Even when treatments do exist their efficacy is often in question. A recent report concluded that 85% of medical and surgical treatments have never been properly tested.

Modern clinicians may use scientific techniques but in the way that they treat their patients they are still quacks and charlatans, loyal to existing and unproven ideas which are profitable and resistant to new techniques and technologies which may be proven and effective.

The fact that a doctor may use a scientific instrument in his work does not make him a scientist - any more than a typist who uses a word processor is a computer scientist. The scientific technology available to doctors may be magnificent but the problem is that the application of the scientific technology is crude, untested and unscientific.

Modern physicians and surgeons do not see the human mind and the human body as a single entity (which is why the medical profession has been slow to embrace the principles of holistic medicine and doubly incompetent in its attempts to deal with stress-related disorders) and they rely more on hopes and assumptions than on evidence and objective clinical experience. The modern clinician is as narrow-minded, and as influenced by his personal experiences and interpretations as was his predecessor 2,000 years ago.

Most patients probably assume that when a doctor proposes to use an established treatment to conquer a disease he will be using a treatment which has been tested, examined and proven. But this is not the case. *The British Medical Journal* in October 1991 carried an editorial reporting that there are `perhaps 30,000 biomedical journals in the world, and they have grown steadily by 7% a year since the 17th century.' The editorial also reported that: `only about 15% of medical interventions are supported by solid scientific evidence' and `only 1% of the articles in medical journals are scientifically sound'. Nothing has improved since then.

What sort of science is that? How can doctors possibly regard themselves as practising a science when six out of seven treatment regimes are unsupported by scientific evidence and when 99% of the articles upon which clinical decisions are based are scientifically unsound? How can doctors regard themselves as scientists when it is known that a kind, compassionate doctor can have a healing rate 50% better than his crueller colleagues - simply because patients respond better to his remedies? How can doctors regard medicine as a science when it has been proven many times that at least a third of patients will get better if given a placebo? How can doctors regard medicine as a science when it is known that a large proportion of patients expecting to have heart surgery will get better if they are merely given a scar on their chests and told that they have had an operation?

Medicine is no science. It's an art. Mysticism.

But these days it is polluted by business. And money.

The savage truth is that most medical research is organised, paid for, commissioned or subsidised by the drug industry. This type of research is designed, quite simply, to find evidence showing a new product is of commercial value. The companies which commission such research are not terribly bothered about evidence; what they are looking for are conclusions which will enable them to sell their product. Drug company sponsored research is done more to get good reviews than to find out the truth.

A study published in the *Journal of the American Medical Association* found that one in five researchers in the life sciences had delayed publication of their results, or had not published them at all, because of their relations with business firms. Whenever I have accused scientists of being prejudiced and `bought' because of their allegiance to their corporate paymasters the answer has invariably been the same: `Everyone does it. There isn't a scientist in the world who hasn't taken corporate money.' This is probably true - and is one explanation for the fact that many allegedly independent Government bodies are almost always packed with men and women who work for (or have taken fees from) the large corporations their Government body is supposed to be policing.

It is also a fact that most of the doctors and scientists writing articles, papers and reviews for medical and scientific journals have received money, grants and freebies from drug, chemical or food companies. (It is also worth remembering that many allegedly and apparently independent journals accept corporate advertising and some accept payment in return for running articles.)

The absence of scientific evidence supporting medical practices is apparent in all areas of medicine.

With a very few exceptions there are no certainties in medicine. The treatment a patient gets will depend more on chance and the doctor's personal prejudices than on science. The unexpected seems to happen so often that it really ought to be expected and the likelihood of a doctor accurately predicting the outcome of a disease is often no more than 50:50.

Even in these days of apparently high technology medicine there are almost endless variations in the treatments preferred by differing doctors. Doctors offer different prescriptions for exactly the same symptoms; they keep patients in hospital for vastly different lengths of time, and they perform different operations on patients with apparently identical problems.

There is, indeed, ample evidence now available to show that the type of treatment a patient gets when he visits a doctor will depend not so much on the symptoms he describes but on the doctor he consults - and where that doctor practises. And yet most doctors in practice seem to be convinced that their treatment methods are beyond question. Many GPs and hospital doctors announce their decisions as though they are carved on stone.

Today's research is largely controlled by and for the pharmaceutical industry. Doctors are unquestioning. Most don't read original papers (and couldn't read between the lines or assess papers accurately even if they did). The majority obtain 99% of their information from two biased and thoroughly unreliable sources: drug companies and the Government. No one bothers to look for evidence that chemotherapy, radiotherapy and vaccination actually work. Since there isn't any this is fortunate and convenient.

Young doctors are told that what they are taught are facts. And they are taught (and then believe) that medicine is a science. Outside the anatomy room and, possibly, the physiology laboratory, there are no facts in medicine. The gaps in our knowledge about the body (when well and when sick) are far greater than the extent of our knowing. Medicine is not a science. It is an art and a craft. With a smidgen of science stuck on the side. Economics, psychiatry and psychology are all pseudosciences with no more relation to real science than astrology or iridology. Medicine is somewhere in between real science and economics. But it isn't a science.

Doctors like to be thought of as scientists because it contributes to their aura of infallibility. Drug companies like to think that doctors are scientists because it encourages patients to have faith in the remedies they produce. And research doctors like to pretend that they are scientists because it makes it easier for them to obtain grants and to tell convincing stories to the media. Modern medical scientists decide on a commercially acceptable solution and then select the facts which support the solution they have selected. That's not science: it's propaganda.

10. Most Research Is Useless

The medical establishment frequently attacks alternative medicine (and seeks to have it banned) on the grounds that no decent research has been done to support the claims made by different practitioners. If that is going to be the new, serious criterion for deciding whether or not a practice should be allowed, much of modern medicine will have to be abandoned including most chemotherapy, more than half of all surgery, all vaccination programmes, nearly all radiotherapy and several billion pounds worth of drugs. And, of course, the whole of psychiatry, without exception. For most of these specialities, and indeed for many more, there has never been any research done to investigate their effectiveness, for others, where research has been done, there is no evidence that they work.

Medicine isn't a science. It is more of a superstition than a science and is closer to astrology than to astronomy. That is why if you visit 12 different doctors with the same set of symptoms you will receive 12 different recommendations. Galileo, Bacon and Vesalius were true scientists who tried to prove, or disprove, their theories dispassionately. Modern medical scientists are more like Paracelsus or Descartes. When doctors say that something is `clinically proven' the phrase is about as meaningful as when used in a toothpaste or hair product advertisement. To the modern medical scientist facts are a nuisance; unsightly blemishes on the medical landscape of prejudices, assumptions and pseudo-scientific fantasies.

In order to dignify their interventions, doctors have traditionally used words (jargon) and tools to give extra power to their mumblings and probings. The first doctors used herbs, trephining, rattles, chants, special bones, ceremonial dances and incantations. Today's doctors use psychotherapy, chemotherapy and radiotherapy. There really isn't a lot more evidence to justify the latest innovations than there is to justify the trephining and incantations.

Most (by which I really do mean more than half) of all research trials conducted today are badly designed and the results are worthless. There are several reasons for this. First, most of those creating and conducting the trials don't understand what they are doing and do not even understand the placebo effect. Second most of the trials are published in journals which rely almost entirely upon drug company advertising. Third, many of the trials are crooked and run on behalf of drug companies. I have provided evidence for this in previous books such as *The Medicine Men, Paper Doctors, Betrayal of Trust, The Health Scandal* and so on.

Despite the drawbacks and failings, billions of pounds are spent every year on medical research programmes. Some research is funded by Governments and multinational corporations but much is funded by charities - which obtain their money through legacies, street collections and the profits from high street shops.

Much of the research which is done is designed to find `magic bullet' style cures. For example, organisations which claim that their purpose is to combat cancer will probably spend a high proportion of their annual research budget on looking for a generic cure for cancer. They usually seem to expect that the `cure' will be a drug.

Hardly any of the billions spent on research is spent on identifying methods to keep people healthy and prevent disease developing, establishing links which would make prevention more scientific, or publicising and promoting information about the maintenance of good health.

This massive, almost universal, international concentration of effort on a search for `magic bullet' drug cures isn't difficult to explain: the reason is that much of the research which is done by organisations performing medical research is co-funded by drug companies, or done on their behalf or with their cooperation and support. Drug companies obviously have a vested interest in the search for a `magic bullet' cure which can be marketed around the world. You will not be surprised to hear that drug companies don't have a great deal of time for treatment programmes which involve a change of diet - and they don't have much time for teaching people how to stay healthy or avoid illness. (It is not surprising that doctors, whose postgraduate medical education is largely paid for or orchestrated by the pharmaceutical industry, are similarly narrow-minded and although some, who earn a living with the knife, may favour surgery over drug therapy, the vast majority of practising doctors believe that the only way to fight illness is with the pen and the prescription pad.)

And it is this link to the drug industry which probably explains why so much of the research which is done involves experiments on animals (even though, as I have shown many times, such research is of absolutely no use to human beings). Indeed, one of the main reasons why the cancer industry has failed so miserably is because it has concentrated too much of its massive effort on animal experiments. Millions of pounds have, for example, been spent on giving cancer to animals - when it has for years been widely appreciated that the cancers animals get are quite different to the cancers people get. It is hardly surprising that the cancer business has been such a dismal failure.

Animal experiments are cheap, relatively easy to perform, do not require great skills, and tend to produce some sort of result very quickly. Cancer research workers often work together with big drug companies which love animal experiments for their double-edged value. If an experiment on a group of animals shows that a drug does not harm those particular animals then the drug company will use the evidence to ensure that the drug is given a clean bill of health around the world. But if an experiment on a group of animals shows that the drug does harm those particular animals the drug company will ignore the evidence on the grounds that animals are different to people - and that the results are, therefore, of no significance. As the American Committee on Diet, Nutrition and Cancer (of the U.S. National Research Council) pointed out in *Diet, Nutrition and Cancer* (published by the National Academy Press): `animals are not human, and the etiology of the cancers they develop may not duplicate that for cancers in humans.' The United States Surgeon General has pointed out: `an important weakness is that virtually all animal studies test single, genetically uniform (inbred) strains of one or two nonhuman species under highly uniform conditions of diet, temperature, stress, exposure to infectious diseases etc.'.

Cancer researchers frequently claim that if animal experiments are banned they will never be able to find a cure for cancer. The choice, they say to those who dare to question what they do, is simple: the lives of a few animals (since animal researchers around the world kill around 1,000 animals every 30 seconds this is something of an under-statement) or the lives of your children. This crude and, sadly, often effective blackmail (which I have previously described as a form of intellectual terrorism) presupposes that cancer researchers are eventually going to find a `cure' for cancer - indeed, it assumes, quite illogically, that there can ever be a single cure for the 200 quite different diseases which make up the group of illnesses we know as `cancer'. There is no evidence at all to suggest that this is an accurate presupposition.

On the contrary, the evidence clearly shows that animal experiments are a complete waste of time, that animal experiments have never led to any useful breakthroughs and that they are never likely to lead to any useful breakthroughs. Animal experiments are expensive, tediously slow, utterly unreliable and almost unbelievably cruel. (I suspect that most of those who defend animal experiments have never even looked at photographs showing the way animals are treated in laboratories.)

Animals get cancer, it is true, but the cancers they get are quite different to the types of cancer which affect human beings. Moreover, animals respond quite differently to the various types of treatment which are available. The results animal researchers obtain are totally without value. The total uncertainty makes the whole business so misleading that the results are (literally) worse than useless.

Instead of helping doctors find a cure for cancer those scientists who do experiments on animals have held back medical progress and have been responsible for much pain and distress and hundreds of thousands of unnecessary deaths.

For example, a standard test used on rats gives results which can be accurately applied to human beings just 38% of the time. This means that 62% of the time the results obtained through animal experiments are wrong. Since tossing a coin would give a long-term 50% chance of accuracy it would clearly be quicker, more effective, more efficient and cheaper for these scientists to spend their working days sitting around tossing coins to assess the safety of chemicals. (`Yes! Heads! We can give this to patients! No! Tails! Patients can't take that one.') But, in political and financial terms, tossing a coin would certainly not be as useful as using animals. Consider tobacco, for example. The link between tobacco and cancer was identified many years ago by doctors whose observations and research work had involved human patients. But long after doctors had established the link between tobacco and cancer in humans animal researchers were still forcing dogs to smoke and painting tobacco tar on the backs of mice in attempts to show whether or not there was a laboratory link between tobacco and cancer. Politicians who wanted to avoid taking action against the wealthy and big tax paying tobacco companies were able to do so on the grounds that they were still awaiting laboratory confirmation of the link between tobacco and cancer. Decades of vague, inconclusive and contradictory results enabled the world's tobacco industry to keep selling a product which is still responsible for approximately one third of all cancer deaths and which, over the years, must have been responsible for more deaths, disease and misery than any other product ever invented.

Using animals to test new anti-cancer drugs is equally absurd. `Test beds' made of human tissue cells are available. These can be used to test anti-cancer drugs. I cannot see the scientific sense in testing a drug on animals when it can be tested on cells which are identical to those within the patients who will take the drug. (There is, as I have already pointed out, coarse commercial sense in doing such tests on animals. If a test on one species shows that a drug is lethal the test can be repeated on another species, and another, and another until a more promising or acceptable result is obtained. The drug can then be launched worldwide as suitable for human patients.) Animal experiments are useless because animals are completely different to people. According to Dr Irwin Bross, giving evidence to the United States Congress: `conflicting animal results have often delayed and hampered the war on cancer, they have never produced a single, substantial advance either in the prevention or treatment of human cancer.' The medical journal *The Lancet* commented that `since no animal tumour is closely related to a cancer in human beings an agent which is active in the laboratory may well prove useless clinically.'

The whole antivivisection movement was demonised in the 1980s and 1990s by Special Branch and MI5 who had no enemy to justify their massive budgets and had to invent one. They chose antivivisectionists even though they must have known damned well that there was never any real danger from them. The whole anti-vivisection movement was (and is) disorganised and consists largely of little old ladies and teenagers handing out badly printed leaflets on street corners on Saturdays. Nevertheless, the Government gave the whole lunacy official backing and a Home Secretary (Jack Straw) described animal rights activists as terrorists. I suspect that the security forces claimed that animal rights activists were a major threat to the nation simply to justify their expensive, existence. And so, old ladies in brogues and tweeds and teenage vegans in cardboard shoes and thin waterproof jackets became the world's most unlikely and least threatening terrorists. Whenever I spoke at anti-vivisection rallies a police helicopter hovered overhead in an attempt to drown out what I was saying.

I believe that vivisectors provide a perfect example of what psychologists call `confirmatory bias. They collect together all the evidence that supports their thesis and then ignore the evidence that is left - the stuff that doesn't support their belief. If pushed into a corner they delight in confusing the issue in every way they can. They will, for example, claim that they are looking after animals better than ever - and are providing them with bigger, nicer cages. And they have a favourite trick which convinces many people. They produce an individual who has been `cured' by a particular drug and then show evidence that the drug was tested on animals. `There you are,' they say, `the animal experiments saved that person's life.' This is, of course, a perfect nonsense. The truth is that the experiments on animals were pointless, irrelevant and unnecessary and played no part in the development of the drug.

In my book *Betrayal of Trust* I named over 50 drugs known to cause cancer or other serious problems in animals but which are prescribed for humans - on the grounds that animals are different to people. And the vivisectors, who admit that over half of their experiments on animals are unreliable and worthless, also admit that they don't know which of their experiments might be useful. So, they clearly don't ever know which of their experiments might be of value. And if you don't know which experiments are of value then all of them are useless.

Those are the arguments I used when giving evidence at the House of Commons and the House of Lords in London. No one said anything in response. Not a word. Moreover, when the House of Lords committee sent me the evidence offered by Britain's Department of Health in support of vivisection I was able to systematically and logically destroy every shred of their evidence. I proved all their arguments in favour of vivisection to be entirely fallacious and nonsensical. I proved, without any shadow of doubt, that vivisection is worse than useless - it is dangerous. (My demolition of the Government's evidence `supporting' vivisection appears on my website www.vernoncoleman.com)

I confess that I was not terribly impressed by the peers who sat on the House of Lords committee on animals. It was a not unpleasant experience. As a witness I was treated with courtesy. It was like being on trial without the inconvenience of being sent to prison if things go badly. One of the peers was someone called Mary Warnock who wrote a book entitled *Nature and Mortality*. This is what she wrote about the committee in her book: `The reason that this committee is such fun is that it is possible, indeed necessary, to discuss these fundamental issues...Our trip to the United States was enormously enjoyable, and I look back on it as a time of endless laughter.' She concluded: `One way and another, it will be a sad day when `Animals' disappears as an entry in my diary.' She clearly had doubts about the value of the committee: `Whether what we recommend will make any difference to the practices of the Home Office is more than doubtful,' she wrote.

Another point worth making is that there is growing evidence to support the contention that many of today's new and most threatening viral epidemics have been generated by medical scientists working with animals. During the 1960's and 1970's cancer researchers and scientists working for the military on the development of death bugs were developing HIV-like viruses in laboratories. They were using animals in their attempts to develop viral weapons with which opponents could be killed (and their countries destabilised) en masse.

Meanwhile, misled by animal studies which suggested that viruses were responsible for the development of cancer researchers were trying to find an anti-cancer vaccine. They combined viruses which were known to cause cancer in animals in an attempt to create new viruses which they hoped would give them some clues about how viruses caused cancer.

Because of incompetence (a common fault among the mass of second rate scientists around the world who routinely perform experiments on animals) the new viruses have been inadvertently spread through our communities. It has subsequently been shown that it possible for deadly new viruses to jump from animals in laboratories to human researchers.

It is worth remembering that the biggest survey of doctors ever conducted showed that the majority of practising doctors agree that animal experiments are of no value whatsoever to doctors and that patients would suffer fewer side effects if new drugs were tested on human cell and tissue cultures. A few years ago I was President of an organisation of over 1,000 doctors who opposed vivisection. The only time I was interviewed by the British media I was subjected to what I can only describe as a lengthy sneer from a presenter called Melvyn Bragg on a radio programme called *Start the Week*.

Vivisectors are, as a group, ignorant, unthinking entirely selfish people who do as much harm to people as they do to animals. They refuse to discuss or debate what they do but rely on misinformation and propaganda. Statistics for 2010 show that the number of `scientific' experiments performed on animals is now higher than it has been for three decades. The Home Office's figures for 2010 show that 3.7 million `procedures' were carried out on 3.6 million cats, dogs, mice, monkeys, rabbits and other animals.

Sadly, it isn't only vivisectors who do worthless research these days.

The worthlessness of most modern medical research has been well documented since I first raised the issue back in the mid 1970s with my second book (*Paper Doctors*). When I wrote *Paper Doctors* I argued that we did not need any more medical research. 'Our libraries are well stocked with information,' I wrote. 'What we need to do now is to concentrate on how to use all the information we have accumulated. There are many cures sitting on the library shelves which are ignored, neglected, overlooked, unrecognised or forgotten. So much new research material is published every year that not even experts in a specific area of medicine would claim to know everything about their speciality.'

Things have not changed.

I still have little or no respect for the majority of modern researchers. And I am, more than ever, convinced that most modern research is worthless.

But some research is needed. The right research could save millions of lives and improve the health of millions. The trouble is that the sort of research we need isn't being done. We need research (requiring careful observation and good record keeping - two historically fundamental foundation stones of good research work) which assesses the value of modern therapies and which examines the link between causes and disease. Sadly, the modern research industry seems to believe that if an experiment isn't done by men and women in white coats and isn't performed in a laboratory, it isn't worth doing.

We also need to stop duplicating research. Even today it is almost impossible to be absolutely certain about whether or not research in a specific area has or has not been done. Research is often duplicated because researchers in one part of the world don't know precisely what has been done (or is being done) in other parts of the world. For decades (since the publication of my book *Paper Doctors*) I have been campaigning (in vain, I fear) for the development of a single, comprehensive research database containing details of every piece of research - whether orthodox or complementary - conducted anywhere in the world.

And how much more research do we really need? If we applied what we already know (and did it effectively and thoroughly) then we would all be much better off. I made this point in *Paper Doctors* in 1977. But ever since then researchers have continued to accumulate knowledge far faster than doctors have been able to apply what has been learned.

11. Original Thinking Is Suppressed By The Medical Establishment

There's no room for initiative and originality in modern medicine. On the contrary, both are actively suppressed. Dissent is officially stifled. Medicine today has become rigid, like other forms of science, and original thinking is as unacceptable today as it was in the days when Semmelweiss was vilified. Most people who work in medicine today don't actually think any more. Oh, they think about what shirt or blouse to wear and they think about what new car to buy and they think about the money they can make but they don't really think about basic, fundamental, important stuff. They don't think about what they are doing with their lives, or why they are doing it or whether it is what they dreamt of doing when they joined the healing profession.

The medical establishment has never been enthusiastic about new ideas. After all, the medical establishment stoutly rejected anaesthesia and the principles of antisepsis and the brave physicians who promoted such ideas had to cope with rejection, cynicism and oppression.

Over the centuries, just about every major advance in medicine has come as a result of the work of eccentric, passionate, determined unclubbables who have fought the establishment and who would today almost certainly fail the newly introduced registration, licensing and revalidation procedures designed to ensure that only doctors who obey every rule of the establishment are allowed to practice medicine.

It is a fact of life that advantageous changes to society happen only through the determined work of unreasonable men. Great things happen only when enough unreasonable men care and are brave enough to be unreasonable in public. Just about all great discoveries in history have been made by people who weren't recognised by their peers before they made their discoveries and often weren't recognised for years afterwards either. When I was writing my book *The 100 Greatest Englishmen and Englishwomen* I was initially astonished at the number of great people who spent at least part of their lives in prison. The explanation, of course, is that many great men and women and almost all original thinkers are, by their very nature, intrinsically rebellious and therefore especially likely to get into trouble with the authorities. And, after all, no one ever did great things by agreeing with the establishment; no one ever changed things for the better without having original ideas. And original ideas are always, almost by definition, an anathema to the establishment. All great innovations, inventions, ideas and developments come from crazy, neurotic people. They may be a little bit or a hell of a lot crazy but they are all crazy. They may be neurotic or psychotic but they certainly aren't boring, sensible or entirely stable. All original and creative people live outside society (and only rarely, and usually towards the end of their careers, do they become members of the establishment); they are, by nature, outsiders. Great advances are never made by people who would be voted into office, made head girl or put in charge of the milk.

There has been woefully little really original thinking in medicine in recent years. This is partly because medical education discourages original thinking, the medical press suppresses original writing and the medical establishment outlaws original thinkers. All real progress is made as a result of observation and deduction but these skills are not valued today. It is, therefore, hardly surprising that there have been very few medical breakthroughs and hardly any bright ideas. Controversy is suppressed and obvious truths ignored for fear of upsetting politicians or some Government protected industry. It is hardly surprising that for years every surgeon `knew' that the best treatment for breast cancer was radical mastectomy, even though there was never any evidence to prove that this was the case. (There are still thousands of surgeons performing radical mastectomies and countless thousands of women having their breasts sawn off unnecessarily.) Worthless, barbaric, dangerous treatments are often followed with great enthusiasm for decades after they have been shown to be utterly wrong-headed. Back in the 19th century surgeons made fortunes by chopping out bits of bowel. Today, surgeons `treat' obesity by stapling stomachs, wiring up jaws and chopping out lengths of bowel.

The doctors who have made the greatest contributions to health care have invariably been attacked, scorned and imprisoned. And today things are worse than they have ever been. Anyone who dares to question today's medical establishment will be suppressed rather than just ignored. History shows that great and useful medical discoveries are invariably made by outsiders; doctors and scientists operating outside the cosy world dominated and controlled by back scratching establishment flunkeys. But in the past such outsiders did at least have a chance to make their contributions. They were reviled and ignored and shut out from polite society but (with surprisingly few exceptions) they were not silenced in the way that original thinkers are silenced today.

Our problem is that the medical establishment was bought by the drug industry decades ago. Today there is no room for initiative and originality and both are actively suppressed. Dissent is officially stifled. The great men of medicine, Snow, Semmelweiss, Lister and so on. would not have survived in today's environment. Anyone who studies medical history can see that the significant developments always come from free thinkers outside the system. Today, more than ever, the free thinkers outside the system are silenced. They will doubtless be defrocked when the new rules of revalidation are introduced to protect the establishment and the pharmaceutical industry.

Traditionally, the medical establishment has quite a record of supporting the wrong view. Over the centuries, if the medical establishment has agreed on something then it has probably been wrong. Today, the power of the establishment to suppress original thought makes things a thousand times worse. Existing therapies which are dangerous, ineffective and even lethal are protected. Tranquillisers and antibiotics are wildly overprescribed but nothing is done to stop the overprescribing. Patients are routinely dispatched to profitable screening clinics which do far more harm than good. Vaccines are injected by the lorry load and children are paralysed and killed by the classroom. Animals are slaughtered in laboratories which are used to preserve the profitability of the drug industry at the expense of patients. Critics are silenced. Eyes are closed to the dangers of genetic engineering and the deteriorating quality of our food supplies. The potential advantages of alternative remedies are dismissed out of hand simply because they might threaten the profitability of the industry which now owns what used to be a profession.

As I explained in *How To Stop Your Doctor Killing You* it has been proven without doubt that most heart surgery is unnecessary. A sensible regime of diet, exercise and stress reduction can reverse the problems now regarded as indications for surgery. But the establishment continues to promote surgery because it is enormously profitable.

New, innovative, safe and effective ways of dealing with diabetes are ignored, suppressed even, because they threaten corporate and professional profitability.

Doctors don't bother looking at scientific evidence any more. It tends to get in the way of profits. The dangers of electricity, mobile telephones and prescription drug contaminated drinking water are all ignored because these threats may prove a financial embarrassment to other parts of the establishment. Powerful evidence proving that all these are real health problems, responsible for many thousands of deaths a year, is suppressed without hesitation.

Iconoclasts are never popular. The people who own and worship the icons don't much care for them being smashed. And these days the icon owners have all the power and most of the money. They control the politicians, the legislature and the media.

Even the media have been bought and are now controlled by the self-serving, self-protecting establishment. It is not, I suspect, widely known but the experts who appear on television and radio, offering apparently independent advice, are usually (nearly always) paid for or subsidised by an industry, and their testimony and advice is, therefore, neither reliable nor consequential. This is as true of medical experts as it is of experts in almost all other fields. The rent-a-quote experts are popular with the media because since they are already being paid by their sponsors they do not ask to be paid for their broadcast appearances. In the days when I was not banned from radio and television I remember contributing to a programme about genetic engineering. Half-way through the programme I asked the other participants, one by one, if they were connected with the genetic engineering industry. Every single one of them admitted that they were being paid by the industry. 'Everyone with an interest in this subject is employed in the industry,' argued one defiant and defensive 'expert'.

The same thing has been prevalent in print media for decades. Much of what is published in the press is placed there by public relations spokesmen and corporate lobbyists. Newspapers and magazines love this material because it comes to them entirely free of charge. Years ago I used to write a weekly, syndicated column which was published in scores of local newspapers. The column was popular with readers (who often wrote and told me that they appreciated my honesty) but not popular with drug companies or the medical establishment (the two are pretty well indistinguishable) and as the months and years went by I was sacked by one newspaper after another and replaced by a variety of doctors (employed either by one of the large drug companies or by the Government) whose sole advantage was that they were all prepared to work for no fee. I remember once asking my agent why we could not compete. 'I can cut your fee,' he said. 'But we're competing with people who work for nothing and it's difficult to make a living when your fee is nothing.'

Over the last few years it has become increasingly clear that bankers, lawyers and politicians have all betrayed us. Despite my best efforts, the public has not yet realised that doctors have betrayed us too. And it will, perhaps, be some time before people realise that whereas politicians, lawyers and bankers have merely impoverished us, doctors have killed our relatives, our friends and our neighbours, have enriched themselves through their legalised slaughter and will most probably kill us too - largely through their determined support of high technology medicine and the pharmaceutical industry.

My theories of bodypower (described in my book *Bodypower* and to the annoyance of the medical establishment now proven to be accurate, sensible and economical) have been attacked and suppressed simply because they are accurate, sensible and economical. How can medical professionals make money out of a system which relies upon allowing the human body to heal itself? (Just the other day I read about a woman who had a baby which refused to take milk from her right breast. The baby would only take milk from the woman's left breast. The woman went to see her doctor who found a lump in the right breast. That's a beautiful example of bodypower. But how can medical professionals make money out of accepting the wisdom of the human body?)

The solutions modern doctors come up with, and the research results they produce, are rarely original or creative or effective. They simply follow the party lines. The majority of today's researchers are unimaginative and incompetent and know that if they want to receive the best grants they must never question the effectiveness of the medical establishment. Most important of all, they must always worship at the shrine dedicated to the pharmaceutical industry.

The Government (encouraged by the fascist arch-enemy of all goodness, the European Union) spends vast amounts of our money creating illness and causing profitable epidemics. The politicians use public money to encourage meat eating - even though they know that meat is now the biggest cause of cancer in the western world. (Politicians who talk about `climate change' and `global warming' but who promote meat eating are Olympic class hypocrites but that is another story.) Politicians prevent people from finding out the truths about the food they buy. They allow advertising that is as manipulative as it is dishonest. And then they throw up their hands in astonishment as the incidence of heart disease, cancer and obesity all rocket. Our present system actively encourages ill health.

In every country where health care is controlled or regulated by the Government, politicians constantly tinker with the administration of health care but what we really need is a reform of our entire approach to life and health. We need a physical revolution, a mental revolution and a spiritual revolution. None of these is likely to come from the medical establishment.

In fact, the modern medical establishment has made enormous and hugely devastating errors in recent years. The medical establishment was dangerously (and now provably) wrong about AIDS. The medical establishment was dangerously (and now provably) complacent about the dangers of overprescribing tranquillisers. For years the establishment ignored the link between tobacco and cancer. For years I was vilified whenever I argued that there was a link between stress and high blood pressure. (My book *Stress Control*, published in the 1970s, was one of the first publications to draw attention to the importance of stress as a cause of illness. I pointed out that nine out of ten modern illnesses are caused, or made worse, by stress. Severe stress can cause extraordinary physical problems. It is, for example, possible for stress to produce a form of dwarfism in children.)

The medical establishment, which long ago sold out to any industry prepared to pay a decent price, always goes along with whatever is convenient and profitable and always opposes evidence which threatens the commercial status quo. Money may not be able to buy you love but it can buy you a whole damned profession. Today's medical profession has oodles of cash but no principles.

These days doctors only get to read and hear what the drug industry wants them to read and hear. Anything controversial, anything questioning the status quo, must be suppressed.

A year or two ago I was invited to speak at a new conference in London. The conference was, I was told, intended to tackle the subject of medication errors and adverse reactions to prescribed drugs. The company organising the conference was called PasTest. `For over 30 years PasTest has been providing medical education to professionals within the NHS,' they told me. `Building on our commitment to quality in medical and healthcare education, PasTest is creating a range of healthcare events which focus on the professional development of clinicians and managers who are working together to deliver healthcare services for the UK. Our aim is to provide a means for those who are in a position to improve services on both national and regional levels. The topics covered by our conferences are embraced within policy, best practice, case study, clinical management and evidence based practice. PasTest endeavours to source the best speakers who will engage audiences with balanced, relevant and thought-provoking programmes. PasTest has proven in the past that by using thorough investigative research and keeping up-to-date with advances in healthcare and medical practice, a premium educational event can be achieved.'

I was delighted. Iatrogenesis (doctor-induced disease) is something of a speciality of mine. I have written numerous books and articles on the subject. My campaigns have resulted in more drugs being banned or controlled than anyone else's.

In addition to my speaking at the conference the organisers wanted me to help them decide on the final programme. I thought the conference was an important one and would give me a good opportunity to tell medical staff and administrators the truth. I signed a contract.

PasTest wrote to confirm my appointment as a consultant and speaker for the PasTest Conference Division. And then there was silence. My office repeatedly asked for details of when and where the conference was being held.

Silence.

Eventually a programme for the event appeared on the Internet. Curiously, my name was not on the list of speakers.

Here is part of the blurb promoting the conference:

'Against a background of increasing media coverage into the number of UK patients who are either becoming ill or dying due to adverse reactions to medication our conference aims to explain the current strategies to avoid adverse drug reactions and what can be done to educate patients.'

Putting the blame on patients for problems caused by prescription drugs is brilliant. Most drug related problems are caused by the stupidity of doctors not the ignorance of patients. If the aim is to educate patients on how best to avoid prescription drug problems the advice would be simple: 'Don't trust doctors.'

The promotion for the conference claims that 'It is estimated errors in medication...account for 4% of hospital bed capacity.' And that prescription drug problems 'reportedly kill up to 10,000 people a year in the UK'. As I would have shown (had I not been banned from the conference) these figures are absurdly low.

The list of speakers included a variety of people I had never heard of including one speaker representing The Association of the British Pharmaceutical Industry and another representing the Medicines and Healthcare Products Regulatory Agency.

Delegates representing the NHS were expected to pay Ł250 plus VAT (Ł293.75) to attend the event. Delegates whose Trust would be funding the cost were asked to apply for a Health Authority Approval form.

So why was I apparently banned from this conference?

This is what PasTest said when we asked them: 'certain parties felt that he (Vernon Coleman) was too controversial to speak and as a result would not attend.'

Could that, I wonder, be the drug industry? Is the drug industry now deciding whom they will allow to speak to doctors and NHS staff on the problems caused by prescription drugs? If I was banned at the behest of the drug industry do NHS bosses know that people attending such conferences will only hear speakers approved by the drug industry and that speakers telling the truth will be banned? (I think it is safe to assume that I won't be invited to speak at any more conferences for NHS staff.)

If I was banned at the behest of the medical profession why are doctors frightened of the truth? (If they think my views are wrong they would surely be happy for me to appear so that they could counter my arguments.)

I could not, of course, be banned by the NHS itself. Why would the NHS not want its employees to know the truth about drug related problems?

Why are people who had me banned so frightened of what I would say? It can surely only be because they know that I would have caused embarrassment by telling the truth.

The scary bottom line is that the NHS paid to send delegates to a conference where someone representing the drug industry spoke to them on drug safety. But I was banned.

Details of the ban were sent to every national and major local newspaper in Britain. None reported it. I sent details of the ban to numerous politicians. None were interested. And yet, the ban seemed to me to strike at the very heart of the nature of the NHS. If health service employees are not allowed to listen to anyone offering ideas which do not fit into the drug company/medical establishment official line what hope is there that patients will be provided with the most appropriate medical care?

The question is this: If the drug companies believe I am wrong why don't they let me speak and then explain why I am wrong? The unavoidable answer is that they know my criticisms of the profession and the industry are accurate and unanswerable.

And the drug industry and the medical profession are, today, inseparable. Today's medical schools teach half truths; they never teach students how to think or criticise the system. (What system is going to teach people to question itself?). Students are educated by rote; taught in the way that dogs are taught tricks. Wisdom is a disadvantage. Common sense is eradicated. Young doctors are incapable of making informed decisions and that suits the pharmaceutical industry just fine. If you don't question perceived notions then how do you ever learn? How does a profession ever progress? Young doctors are never exposed to the truth or to the questioning of `accepted' beliefs or to proper debate (e.g. with people like me). So medical schools churn out platoons of unquestioning prescription signing zombies. Originality is a dirty word.

Good doctors need insight, imagination and intuition and the capacity to make diagnostic leaps; sideways if necessary. Good doctors need to be able to observe and they need to be able to think. Great discoveries are invariably made by outsiders and mavericks. Such skills are not simply not encouraged; they are now not allowed. As a result the medical profession is packed with drudges, unthinking, too frightened of losing their jobs to show any spirit

Doctors do not have the courage to question the establishment or to have original ideas because they are employed and like all other employees they are frightened of losing their jobs. Moreover, NHS doctors are employed by the Government; they are civil servants. Today's doctors are bought, body, mind and soul, and do not have the courage to stand up for whatever principles they might have. They do not dare disagree with their administrative bosses because they are hired hands. They do not dare stick up for their patients because they live in fear of bureaucratic censure. And so they vaccinate, and they perform unnecessary operations and they prescribe drugs which they should know are unsafe. Tonsils and lengths of intestine are ripped out by surgeons who don't seem to have the foggiest notion of the harm they are doing. Healthy breasts are slashed off unnecessarily.

Doctors do not have the courage to stand up for their patients because they have lost their independence; they are simply civil servants; they have sold their souls for a fat salary, short working hours and a wonderful pension. They are so beholden to their employers that they dare not even stand up to bullying, they dare not even speak out when they see things happening which they know, in their hearts, are wrong. Their spirits have curdled.

The modern medical establishment elevates its official beliefs into an orthodoxy, always suggesting that they are right because they are, well, right and that the absence of evidence is not to be allowed to interfere with the acceptance of their conclusions. This is tabloid science.

For example, the supporters of vaccination deal with opposition not by debate but by denouncing anyone who disagrees. It's the same approach as is used by climate change advocates. Critics are demonised as flat-earthers or holocaust deniers or accused of being in the pay of someone. The only debate allowed is about how big a problem we have created - we are never allowed to discuss whether climate change is man-made because that is 'fact'. Anyone who disagrees is a dangerous heretic - to be excluded from all debates, and condemned and isolated.

Back in the 1980s I dared to question the argument that AIDS would kill us all. The medical establishment announced gravely that by the year 2000 we would all be touched by AIDS. I was roundly attacked by the profession, the politicians and the media by questioning the logic of these claims and by daring to introduce fact based arguments into the arena.

Science has been hijacked by politically correct lobbyists. Dissenters, daring to question the new orthodoxy of the group-think obsessionals, are guilty of thought crime and to be vilified and suppressed. Group think unoriginality oppresses and suppresses.

Now, new regulatory licensing schemes for doctors in the UK mean that practising doctors will in future have to be revalidated by a senior doctor who will make recommendations about their fitness to practice. It seems to me likely that this will mean that any doctor who does not stick to the rules will be refused a licence and prevented from practising.

Just about every significant doctor in history, from Semmelweiss to Snow, would have failed the licensing scheme as planned and I have absolutely no doubt that, for example, the new system will ensure that any doctor who opposes, questions or in any way criticises vaccination will be removed from the medical register before you can say 'scientific bigotry'.

The chances of anyone questioning the medical establishment in the future will be close to non-existent. It is today more dangerous for a doctor to be ahead of his time (which is to say, critical of well-established but ill-advised and dangerously nonsensical medical practices) than it is for him to be behind his time. The doctor who dares to criticise the acknowledged mainstream is still a dangerous heretic who must be crushed.

Over the last four decades I have made many forecasts about medical hazards. Most have already been proved entirely accurate. But accuracy is no defence against ridicule, abuse, scorn and scepticism; indeed, since being correct makes the authoritarians fearful, the ridicule, abuse, scorn and scepticism are enhanced.

12. Most Doctors Are Addicted To Prescribing

Most doctors are obsessed with drug therapy. Many don't seem to have heard of the many effective non-drug solutions which now exist. If it doesn't come in a blister pack and isn't packaged by one of the world's big drug companies they don't believe it can possibly work.

The big mistake most doctors make is to assume that drug companies are in business because they want to make sick people well again. That is a big, big mistake. The drug companies make drugs. That is what they do. But they make drugs so that they can make a profit. (And that they do very well - better, indeed, than any other industry.) Drug companies do not exist to help patients get better. They exist solely to make profits - they use sickness as a route to profit. And, to be frank, why should we expect them to be in business for any other reason?

Motor car companies aren't in business because they want to help people move around. They are in business because they think they can make a profit out of selling cars. Supermarkets aren't in business because they want to make shopping easier and cheaper. They are in business to make a profit. Arms companies don't make bombs and landmines because they want to help small, threatened countries defend themselves against aggressive neighbours. They make bombs and landmines because they can make big profits out of selling them.

I don't hate drug companies but I do think we need to regard them with great scepticism for they are (together with the food and tobacco industries) one of the three major modern threats to human health.

Doctors simply do not understand any of this. They wrongly assume that the drug companies have interests which match the interests of their patients.

This is silly.

If doctors thought this through they would realise that patients and drug companies have diametrically opposed interests. The patient wants to get better. But the drug company will make bigger profits if the patient remains ill - and continues to need to take drugs.

But either through collective stupidity or through naivety (or because they like being bribed by drug companies) doctors like to believe that drug companies exist for the good of mankind.

Doctors should regard drug companies with caution and they should keep their relationship with them at arms length. They should regard drug companies as providing just one group of possible remedies. But collectively doctors have behaved pretty stupidly. They have sold out to the drug industry and they have (as I pointed out over a third of a century ago) become little more than a marketing arm of the world's most profitable industry.

Drug companies have, not surprisingly, welcomed and taken advantage of the medical profession's collective stupidity (and/or naivety). They have virtually taken over postgraduate medical education. Their advertising dominates medical journals. And as a result most doctors (not just the bad ones) are obsessed with drugs because they simply aren't aware that there are other ways to deal with health problems.

In the last century the practice of medicine has become no more than an adjunct to the pharmaceutical industry and the other parts of the huge, powerful and immensely profitable health care industry.

Medicine is no longer an independent profession.

Doctors are now no more dedicated to the saving of lives and the improvement of patients' welfare than are the thousands of drug company salesmen and marketing men. Doctors have become nothing more than a link connecting the pharmaceutical industry to the consumer.

It is not difficult to see why the drug industry behaves in such a ruthless manner. The profits to be made out of selling drugs are phenomenal. It is not at all uncommon for a drug company to sell several hundred million dollars worth of one product in a year. Companies can make over 90 pence pure profit for every one pound's worth of a drug that they sell. The raw materials for a drug may cost less than $100 a kilo. Turning the raw materials into 100,000 pills and packing them may take the total cost to $1000. The retail price for 100,000 pills may be over $100,000. The only other internationally sold product that can compare for profitability is cocaine.

Drug companies frequently make minimum annual profits of between 30% and 50% on their capital employed. These profits, incidentally, come after the massive above and below the line payments to doctors.

Nor are profits likely to drop because the number of drugs doctors prescribe does not seem to be slowing down. A recent survey of over 2,000 patients admitted to hospital showed that within a ten year period the number of drugs prescribed per patient had shown an increase of almost 50%. Today it is hard to avoid the conclusion that medicine is run for the benefit of large drug companies which make fortunes out of persuading gullible doctors to prescribe useless drugs. Persuading ill-informed doctors (and ignorant nurses who have demanded and been given the authority to prescribe) to prescribe their wretched products is a highly profitable business.

The importance of drug therapy, and the reverence with which drugs are regarded by doctors and nurses, is perhaps best seen in modern rural health centres where doctors dispense as well as prescribe and where the dispensing counter where patients exchange their prescription slips for drugs is rather akin to a high altar. The modern consultation is, too often, a simple, uncomplicated, thoughtless three part process. First, the patient visits the doctor and reports his or her symptoms. Second, the doctor decides which drug (or, more likely, which drugs) will be most appropriate and writes out what he considers to be an appropriate prescription. And, third, the patient takes the prescription to the high priest and has it turned into a bottle of pills, a tube of ointment, an inhaler or whichever form has been deemed appropriate. Doctors are trained and kept up-to-date by and for the pharmaceutical industry. This may sound like hyperbole. It isn't. Drug companies pay for a very large part of the education that a doctor receives.

It seems that everyone in modern health care worships at the sterile shrine of the pharmacy. And the whole thing is made infinitely worse by the fact that approximately half of all the prescriptions doctors write are for patients they don't see. Every single day of the working week half a million repeat prescriptions are collected from GP's surgeries - frequently by patients who never needed to be on drugs in the first place. Back in the mid 1980s I pointed out that Britain's huge tranquilliser and sleeping pill addiction problem had been caused largely by the growth in `repeat prescribing'. Nothing has changed. Not long ago a GP was fined for continuing to issue repeat prescriptions for a patient who had died.

Prescription drugs can, and do, save many lives. But prescription drugs are one of the major killers in our modern world. If drugs were only ever prescribed sensibly, and when they were likely to interfere with a potentially life-threatening disease, then the risks associated with their use would be acceptable. But all the evidence shows that doctors do not understand the hazards associated with the drugs they use and frequently prescribe inappropriately and excessively. Many of the deaths associated with drug use are caused by drugs which did not need to be taken.

Patients are given the wrong drug.

Or they are given the wrong dose of the right drug.

Or they are given the right drug by the wrong route (for example, a drug that should be injected into a muscle may be injected directly into the bloodstream).

Experts believe that there is an error roughly one in every eight times when a hospital patient is given a drug.

Since an ordinary hospital patient may receive a dozen different drugs - at different times of the day - the opportunities for error are colossal. In a 300 bed hospital there may be between 300 and 400 medication errors every day! Some of those errors will result in mild discomfort. Some will result in death.

One of the perks of travelling first class on Eurostar is that there's a varied selection of free magazines to choose from at the end of each carriage. I picked up a free copy of the *New Statesman* on Eurostar recently. It's an odd little magazine, every bit as twee as *The Lady, The Spectator, Country Life* and the *Economist.* They all seem to me to be little more than cult newsletters, catering to their own peculiar tribes of prejudiced and bigoted zealots. The *New Statesman* I picked up included a supplement entitled *The people's NHS?* The supplement was published `in collaboration with Pfizer'. Now, Pfizer is of course an international pharmaceutical company. Strange bedfellows. I wonder if anyone at the *New Statesman* knows enough about drug companies to have asked themselves why one of them should agree to help pay for a *New Statesman* publication. The back of the supplement explains that Pfizer and the *New Statesman* aim to bring together leading opinion-formers to explore a range of health issues relevant to policymakers and the electorate alike (are there any health issues not relevant to both?). We are told, moreover, that Pfizer sponsors these events and collaborates with the *New Statesman* to determine the discussion topics. I bet it does. There's a bit of text telling readers that the *New Statesman* has sole editorial responsibility for the content of the supplement. Oh how sweet that is. Dare I point out that one of the contributors just happens to be a senior director of Pfizer. What an amazing coincidence that is. If anyone at the *New Statesman* is interested here's the bottom line: Pfizer sponsors the *New Statesman* events (and helps choose the discussion topics) because the drug companies love the NHS. It is a cash cow of unprecedented size. Always giving. And I don't mind betting that this merry duo of Pfizer and the *New Statesman* never produce anything questioning the whole existence of the NHS, or the dangers produced by modern drugs or question the value of vaccination or vivisection. Drug companies are everywhere these days. It is impossible for two doctors to meet, or a politician and a doctor to discuss health matters or, it seems, a left wing magazine to produce a supplement without a drug company being involved (and usually paying for the smart lunch or dinner afterwards).

There are two large, international drug industries on this planet. One of these two industries makes huge amounts of money out of ruthlessly promoting dangerous and often lethal products. The other drug industry, much smaller, much less profitable and far less ruthless, sells drugs such as cocaine and heroin and is responsible for a relatively small number of deaths. And the *New Statesman* would have been wiser to have an `arrangement' with the second than with the first.

The myth that drug therapy offers the only true solution is now repeated unquestioningly and without hesitation or embarrassment. In America the big drug companies spend $5 billion every year on marketing their drugs and persuading doctors to prescribe them. (In 2004 a company called Astra Zeneca spent $216 million promoting a cholesterol reducing drug called Crestor. That's $4 million more than PepsiCo spent on marketing that year.) In India the average urban doctor is visited by an average of 20 (20!) sales representatives every day. And all this promotion has an effect: it has been shown that doctors who accept lunches, fees or perks from drug companies are more likely to prescribe the companies' products. Doctors who get paid to do research or give a lecture are up to 19 times more likely to request a company's products. When doctors are choosing a drug to prescribe they are led not by scientific principles but by commercial principles. For example, drug companies hand out lots of free pens and notepads. These pens and notepads have the names of drugs printed on them. Drug companies give these away because they know that a doctor will probably prescribe the drugs whose names are on their pens and notepads. That's an appalling truth. In Italy the police asked for almost 5,000 people to be put on trial (including 4,400 doctors and at least 273 employees of a major drug company). The complaint was that the company had spent Ł152 million on sweeteners to doctors and chemists. The sweeteners (it seems silly not to call them bribes) consisted of holidays, cameras, computers and cash.

Not long ago a drug company gave each doctor who wanted one a new fax machine. The drug company paid for a line to be installed and then paid the line rental. Why? So that they could 'stay in touch' with the doctor. And doctors can get free Blackberries and other gadgets too. So that drug companies can keep in touch. Drug companies organise `disease awareness weeks', they sponsor patients associations (which are sometimes little more than drug promoting groups), they send letters to agony columnists (and follow these letters with literature containing an appropriate answer) and they set up apparently independent health sites on the Internet. I frequently receive e-mails from companies wanting to advertise their products on my website. (My website remains free of advertising and sponsorship.) The *British Medical Journal* website - available to the public - contains drug company advertising.

The basic problem is money. The pharmaceutical industry has a lot of it. And doctors want more of it. The result is that the industry has bought the profession (or most of it). When I have spoken to individual doctors I have invariably been able to convince them of the horrors of the present system. But most doctors, even when they have had their eyes opened to what is happening, prefer to close their eyes again. They find it all too alarming and too frightening. They just don't want to know. They don't think we can change anything. And they are frightened of causing trouble because they know that if they cause trouble their careers will be finished. Young doctors are particularly nervous about speaking out. Older doctors are often `bought' and too much in need of the money they can get from the drugs industry to sustain their lifestyles. Millions die and suffer because the medical establishment has sold its soul. If more doctors dared to question the authorities the world would be a very different (healthier and happier) place. The tragedy is that no one in the medical establishment cares much about facts or evidence. They have numerous preconceived ideas - which, by a beautiful coincidence, just happen to fit in with the needs and wants of the drug industry.

The Government and the drug industry controlled medical profession are now even enthusiastic about healthy people taking drugs. There are, for example, around four million people in Britain now taking cholesterol-lowering 'superdrugs'. In July 2008, it was revealed that these drugs might cause problems. Readers of my book *How To Stop Your Doctor Killing You* have been aware of the problems associated with these drugs since 1996. Despite the dangers the cholesterol lowering drugs are widely advertised and promoted - even though I don't believe there is evidence that these drugs are safe or useful enough for such mass consumption.

As drug companies become increasingly aware that curing serious disease is beyond their capability (and, indeed, their desire - for why should drug companies, which make their money out of people being sick, want to make people well?), they spend more and more effort on finding drugs to improve life or performance in some vague way. Profits, not patients, are now the driving force which rule the medical profession's motives, ambitions and actions. Doctors don't seem to care any more. The passion has gone out of medicine.

Medical journals claim that they make researchers disclose their financial links to drug companies when writing about their products. However, I doubt if there are 100 doctors in Britain who can honestly claim that they are not linked in some way to a drug company, have not had a meal off them, or do not have an office full of free pens or a golf bag full of sponsored balls.

When the *LA Times* looked at 36 drug therapy articles published it found that eight had been written by researchers who hadn't disclosed their links to drug companies. I'm surprised they found so few. One study showed that 96% of authors who wrote favourably about calcium channel blocking drugs used for angina and high blood pressure had some sort of financial relationship with the drug company making the drug being discussed and that in only two out of 70 articles did authors divulge their connection. And, as I have shown many times in the past, even Government safety committees are riddled with people who have links to drug companies.

On 22nd February 2011, the Government warned that a large number of patients who are being treated for high blood pressure don't actually have high blood pressure. How this could possibly be described as news is quite beyond me. I first warned that blood pressure was being over treated over 30 years ago. Naturally, I was pilloried for it by the medical establishment and the medical press. But it wasn't a difficult conclusion to draw. As a GP I often acquired new patients who had been given repeat prescriptions for powerful anti-hypertensive therapies for years without ever seeing a doctor. In the early 1970s I was criticised viciously for daring to suggest that blood pressure could often be raised by stress and could, therefore, be brought under control if sufferers learned how to control their stress. Moreover, it is often remarkably easy for people with moderately high blood pressure to bring their blood pressure down simply by making moderate lifestyle changes (losing weight, giving up cigarettes, taking gentle exercise, reducing their exposure to stress and so on.) I have lost count of the number of readers who have followed my advice on this and been able to bring their blood pressure under control. Why does it always take doctors so long to see the obvious? The answer, of course, is that doctors are controlled by drug companies. And drug companies prefer to treat every symptom or sign with drugs - whether it is necessary to do so or not. Today, more than 8.5 million people in the UK are registered as having high blood pressure. All are treated with expensive and dangerous drugs. The Government now says that a quarter of these don't have it. That is a massive under-estimate. At least a half of these do not have high blood pressure - and never had it. Moreover, at least half of the remaining half could control their blood pressure without drug treatment.

Even more scary is the fact that most medical treatments are untried and unproven to be any good at all. The evidence for this apparently provocative claim can be found in books of mine such as *How To Stop Your Doctor Killing You* and *Betrayal of Trust*. Even drug treatments which are well established have still not yet been properly evaluated. For example, doctors still don't know whether a course of antibiotics should be given for five, seven, ten or fourteen days for the best results.

Drugs are wildly overprescribed, both by hospital doctors and by general practitioners. It is now over 30 years since I first exposed the dangers of benzodiazepines and over 20 years since a Tory Government admitted that it had introduced new legislation as a result of my campaign. But still benzodiazepines are overprescribed and still they are prescribed badly, without thought and without awareness of the often disastrous consequences for patients. Vast numbers of other drugs, including antibiotics and painkillers as well as antidepressants, are frequently overprescribed. Vaccines are a major cause of illness and death.

Much of the medical establishment denies all this, of course, and still steadfastly and stubbornly refuses to acknowledge that `alternative' or `complementary' medical techniques have a great deal to offer. Gentle therapies, and gentle practitioners, are deliberately demonised by the drug industry controlled medical establishment. A reader wrote to say that her late husband was a pharmacist for over 60 years. She said that although his daily job was dispensing medicines he always preferred to use natural remedies himself. He was, she said, amazed at the length of time patients were kept on some drugs without any check to find out if they still needed them.

Surprisingly, even universities are now very closely linked to drug companies. Since 1988, British universities have been allowed to exploit the intellectual property they generate. As a result, academics around the world have become multimillionaires through working on new drugs while accepting university salaries. They and the drug companies then make fortunes out of the work done with taxpayers' money. Astonishingly, 45 out of the world's 50 top selling drugs were developed and or tested with taxpayers' money. So many academics have links to drug companies that there are now virtually no independent scientists in Britain. Corruption is embedded and endemic.

The result is that the emphasis during medical training is far too much on profit and far too much on drug therapy. Most medical schools don't bother to teach students anything about alternative therapies. Doctors are taught nothing about nutrition or relaxation. Alternative remedies are sneered at and often banned because of the power of the big drug companies. An astonishing 95% of malaria victims can be cured within three days with a few tablets made with an extract from the leaves of the sweet-wormwood weed. This medicine was used virtually to rid Vietnam of malaria in the 1990s. Western attempts to deal with malaria have been an abject and scandalous failure. The death rate from malaria has continued to climb and the disease is one of the world's worst killers. The WHO approved the extract from sweet-wormwood in 2001 but the big American drug companies actively and successfully opposed its use. The problem, for them, is that the raw materials come from China and no American company owns a patent on the product. So, in Africa around 3,000 children die every day from malaria. And yet, although they were keen to prevent a non-patented product being made available, the drug companies pay very little attention to malaria. Orthodox doctors routinely lie about the value of alternative medicines. Anyone who says that alternative therapy never works for cancer, for example, is either very stupid, a sadist or simply woefully ill-informed. Or, perhaps, receiving a large grant or fee from a drug company.

When he writes out a prescription your doctor has to rely upon the honesty and integrity of the drug company making the product he is prescribing. And since most drug companies do not operate in an honest way that is a fundamental error of trust which can lead to many problems. You suffer from his trust in the drug company. To that you must add the fact that all patients are individual and different. A drug which has proved effective and safe when given to 99 or 999 patients may still prove dangerous and deadly when given to the 100th or the 1000th patient. Every patient who takes a drug - even a well tried drug - is participating in an experiment. Most doctors either do not understand this or they forget it in the heat of daily practice. To make things worse, doctors often prescribe several drugs at once; frequently prescribing two drugs which interact dangerously. The dangers of polypharmacy still fail to be recognised, even though interactions are common and can be deadly.

On 24th June 2011 the British press reported that researchers had warned doctors that mixtures of common prescription drugs could kill and might exacerbate serious health problems such as dementia. It was announced in the *Daily Telegraph* that the new research `shows for the first time that mixing drugs has a significant impact on a patient's chance of death'.

However, I have been warning for many years that drug interactions are dangerous and deadly. In my book *The Medicine Men* (first published in 1975) I wrote: `It is the problem of drug interactions which is likely to cause most controversy in the future. There are many possibilities. Metabolism of one drug may affect another. Drugs may react chemically together within the body and excretory rates may be modified with devastating results. Patent medicines and even foodstuffs may react.'

I then spent several pages of the book explaining why drug interactions were so potentially dangerous.

That was in 1975. But neither doctors nor journalists take much notice of history - especially when it is inconvenient.

Sadly, tragically, doctors have become so used to doing what they are told by the industry that they have become accustomed to prescribing pills for every problem. They have lost the breadth of vision to enable them to see opportunities for cure outside the traditional range of pharmacological opportunities.

The drug industry has convinced doctors that everyone they see must need a drug and that there is a pill for every ill. The majority of doctors might as well be employed directly by the drug companies as pretend to be independent, authoritative scientists. They prescribe what they are told to prescribe in exactly the same way that the drug company representatives promote what they are told to promote.

The modern doctor would like to be regarded as a mystical healer; that, indeed, is how he probably sees himself in his dreams. But in reality the modern doctor is little more than a drug company employee; pushing the latest line in wonder drugs with evangelical enthusiasm, never daring to criticise or to question the promotional material he is shown, grasping his free pen, golf ball or umbrella and wearily handing out the latest wonder drug until it is superseded by another wonder drug and imagining that by prescribing the latest new drug he is remaining on the frontiers of science and helping to push back the barriers of ignorance. How many know, I wonder, that new drugs are tested and licensed for safety (in a vague, entirely satisfactory sort of way it has to be said) but not for effectiveness.

The fact that the medical profession is dominated and controlled by the pharmaceutical industry would not matter so much if the drug industry were honest, responsible and ethical. But it isn't. There is no other industry in the world which is as profitable or as ruthless as the drugs industry.

According to a survey published in the *Annals of Internal Medicine* nearly two thirds of the pharmaceutical advertisements in medical journals were either grossly misleading or downright inaccurate. A total of 109 advertisements from 10 leading medical journals were each reviewed by two doctors and an academic clinical pharmacist. The reviewers used guidelines from the Food and Drug Administration to assess the advertisements. In 30% of cases the independent reviewers disagreed with the advertiser's claim that the drug was the drug of choice. In 44% of cases the reviewers thought that the advertisement would lead to improper prescribing if a doctor had no information about the drug other than that provided in the advertisement.

New diseases are `discovered' all the time. You will excuse my cynicism, and my suspicion that these new diseases are discovered for a reason, when I tell you that most of these new diseases just happen to be enormously profitable. One of the most profitable is a disorder known as COPD (chronic obstructive pulmonary disease) which is actually a relatively new catch all name for a variety of chest disorders including asthma, emphysema and chronic bronchitis. In the bad old days patients with these individual disorders were treated as when treatment was required. Today, the new philosophy seems to be that patients with COPD should take constant medication - whether they actually need it or not.

Another new disease is `isolated systolic hypertension'. Just a few years ago doctors believed that only the diastolic figure was of significance when measuring blood pressure. The systolic, or higher figure, was regarded as of little consequence by itself. And then drug companies noticed that around 80% of all individuals over the age of

65 had normal diastolic pressures but systolic pressures that were high compared with younger patients. And so, surprise, surprise, a new disease came into being - `isolated systolic hypertension' - and it became necessary for doctors to start treating the high systolic pressure.

Occasionally politicians mutter about the obscene levels of drug company profits but the industry is efficient and ruthless and politicians are usually dealt with easily. The truth is that most politicians are, for a variety of reasons, reluctant to interfere with the drug industry. Drug companies provide jobs and pay taxes; in most developed countries they bring in revenue from abroad. Even the least effective drug company should be able to sell its product to developing countries.

But the key factor in the failure of the politicians to control the drug industry is surely that neither politicians nor industrialists are particularly keen to see illness conquered. The drug industry wants to see as many people as possible suffering from long-term, incurable illnesses. The politicians wants to see people die before they become old and dependant. If more money was spent on preventing cancer (around 80% of cancers are preventable and other diseases) then the average life expectancy would go up dramatically and the incidence of disease and disability would fall. But the drug industry doesn't want a healthy nation (it would sell fewer drugs) and the politicians don't want any more people living to an old age because they know that they would not be able to cope with the pension bills they would have to pay. The astonishing truth is that the drug industry needs to keep the voters ill in order to maintain its profits and the politicians want to help them achieve that aim.

The medical establishment, which has sold its soul for pots of gold and which is now controlled by an industry whose primary aim is to maximise the number of sick people in society, rarely criticises the drug industry. Most academic research departments, medical journals and medical associations rely heavily if not exclusively on the drug industry. The drug industry effectively owns the medical establishment.

A reader wrote to me and suggested that if drug companies got their way the official NHS motto would be 'First do not heal'. He is absolutely right. Drug companies do not want patients to be healed. Sick people are profitable. Healthy people are not. Turning people into chronic invalids is far more profitable than curing them.

13. The Unfair Sex

Politicians and bureaucrats who know nothing about anything but regulate everything, decreed, back in 1974, that there must, in future, be the same number of female doctors as there are male doctors. There is no law ruling that there should be as many male nurses, models or ballet dancers as there are female nurses, models or ballet dancers but there is a rule (doubtless originating in some luxurious and expensively furnished office in Brussels) that there must be as many women doctors as there are men doctors.

It was decided that this absurd and extraordinarily sexist law would be enforced by introducing sexual discrimination into medical school selection policies.   As a result, well over half of all new medical students are now female. The aim is not just to produce as many women doctors as male doctors but to make the total number of women doctors equal to the total number of male doctors. Since there have traditionally been far more male doctors than female doctors the changes are being made quickly and dramatically by training more women than men.

This sexist lunacy is destroying medicine as a profession and killing patients by the thousand. Forcing medical schools to take a greater percentage of girls than boys has been disastrous; there are always fewer girls than boys applying and so medical schools have had to take the dregs of the female applications in order to match their quotas. Moreover, there are far fewer women who genuinely want to be doctors - and students who aren't driven by a real vocation make terrible doctors. Naturally, no one dares protest about this obscene and dangerous example of sexual discrimination, despite the fact that it is producing very real problems.

The truth is that the majority of women doctors should be doing something else for a living - nursing, perhaps. Patients - both male and female - would be much better off without them. There is good science behind this apparently politically incorrect argument. It is well-known that accidents rise considerably when a woman is premenstrual. Astonishingly, 93% of crimes committed by women are committed in the premenstrual phase and it is not infrequently argued that women who commit crimes when their hormones are bewildered should not be convicted. Accidents in the home and on the road rise dramatically in that time of the month. Should women be allowed to have positions of authority of responsibility? Doesn't all this make it dangerous to put women in charge of operating theatres, Government departments or police forces? The question should at least be asked. But no one in authority has the guts to ask it. And even if they did no one would have the courage to answer it honestly.

The decree that medical students should be selected not according to vocation or intellect but according to chromosome resulted in massive changes to the whole philosophy of medical care and, allied to the changes in working hours introduced as a result of legislation introduced by the European Union, destroyed the concept of continuity of care. I have no doubt that the insistence that medical schools give preference to women is one of the fundamental reasons for the deterioration in the quality of medical care.

Women doctors want to work part-time; they want to be home when their children come in from school, they want to be there to make tea, they don't want to work at nights or at weekends or on bank holidays. They want to have a year off every time they have a baby. And, of course, they want to have time off when they have 'time of the month' hormone problems. (Much the same thing has happened in Parliament, of course. Female politicians and Ministers don't want to work evenings or weekends.)

Am I the only one to have noticed that medicine is now controlled by women? Most senior nurses are women. Many senior administrative positions are held by women. And new equality laws mean that there are now more women doctors than ever before.

Is it really a coincidence that medical care is in a worse state than ever?

14. Killed By Prescription

Every few months another scandal exposes the dangers of a particular prescription drug: a seemingly safe and widely prescribed drug is found (often more by accident than deliberate research) to have been responsible for hundreds or thousands of deaths and serious injuries. The manufacturer will at first dispute the revelations and will then argue that the 'cost' (the number of deaths and disabilities caused by the drug) was acceptable and an unavoidable risk. The drug may or may not be withdrawn, or the guidelines may be changed slightly. There will be no apologies. There is unlikely to be any compensation. Attempted lawsuits are usually seen off with the help of (highly-paid) expert medical advisors giving evidence on behalf of the company.

But all this is little more than a superficial distraction. The real problem, and the real cause of the endemic problem of iatrogenesis, is the steady drip drip of death and disability caused by hundreds or thousands of widely prescribed prescription drugs which remain on the market.

Doctors believe (because they want to believe it) that drugs are reliable and effective. As long as doctors believe this then they can convince themselves that *they* are reliable and effective and useful. But the truth is that drug making is so crude that Severin Schwan the boss of Roche, the massive and powerful Swiss drugs firm has said: `Drugmaking is so crude that half of all known diseases cannot be treated at all, and the drugs for the other half work properly only half the time and with huge side effects.'

It is this gap between hope and expectation on the one side, and reality on the other, which results in so much danger and so much illness.

The truth, of course, is that all drugs are potentially harmful. There isn't a drug on the planet which can't do harm - and even kill people. It's the risk-benefit relationship which doctors (and patients) ignore. If a doctor gives you a drug without which you will die then the risks are almost inconsequential. But if you don't really need a drug and the drug makes you ill then the risk is unacceptable. Antibiotics save lives. But they also kill people. If you have an infection which might kill you then taking an antibiotic is a good thing. But if you have a viral infection then taking an antibiotic (which might kill you) is pretty stupid. There's no benefit but a lot of risk. Some drugs are potentially useful. All drugs are potentially harmful.

Most people take far too many medicines - without knowing why they are taking them, what the medicine is designed to do, what the side effects might be and what might happen if the drug is not taken. Doctors have created drug dependency among patients. To understand why you have to understand the history of the modern general practitioner. Today's GP is descended from the apothecary. And apothecaries weren't allowed to charge a consultation fee. The only way they could make money was by prescribing and dispensing potions. The business of handing out drugs has become a part of the consultation ritual. When a doctor doesn't have the foggiest idea what to do she reaches for the prescription pad. And, of course, many doctors use the prescription pad as a way to cut short a consultation. Not surprisingly, doctor-induced illness is now a major problem. It may often be easier to end a consultation by handing over a prescription or a medicine. But that doesn't mean that it is the right thing to do. On the contrary, doctors should be more responsible for this. They should educate their patients and they should only prescribe drugs when drugs are essential, useful and likely to do more harm than good.

Sadly, doctors know very little about the medicines they recommend to their patients. Most of the information they have comes directly from the company selling the product - which obviously has a vested interest in promoting the virtues and covering up the defects. As a result of this ignorance four out of every ten patients who visit a doctor and receive a prescription will suffer noticeable, severe or even lethal side effects. If a patient is taking a drug which will help keep him alive then side effects are an acceptable risk. But if a patient is taking a drug he doesn't really need then the risks are unacceptable.

Since the end of the 1970s I have argued that we need an international computerised drug monitoring service - designed to make sure that doctors in one part of the world know when doctors in other countries have spotted problems. Astonishingly, no such system exists. You might imagine that when a drug is withdrawn in one country other countries will take similar action. But you would be wrong. One drug that was officially withdrawn from the market in the USA and France was not officially withdrawn in the UK until five years later.

The myth that we live long and healthy lives thanks to the drug industry and the medical profession has increased our expectations. We no longer expect to fall ill. We expect a magic solution when we fall ill. We don't want to be bothered making any effort to stay healthy because we have been taught to have faith that if we fall ill then the medical men will be able to cure us.

It is widely accepted that the majority of illnesses do not need drug treatment. Most patients who visit a doctor neither want nor expect drug treatment. But at least eight out of ten patients who visit a general practitioner will be given a prescription (though growing numbers of patients do not take the drugs that are prescribed for them). Huge numbers of people in the community are given drugs which have only ever been tested on hospital patients. I think patients should always be aware of the potential side effects of any drug they take (whether they take it for medical, social or recreational reasons). Only when patients know the downside can they make a rational decision about whether the risk in taking a particular drug is worth taking. How many of the patients taking a drug know the full picture? (There is a free list of possible side effects for many of the most popular prescription drugs on my website www.vernoncoleman.com).

Ironically, although we consume greater and greater quantities of medicine than ever before more of us are ill today than at any time in history. On any day you care to choose in just about any developed country you care to mention over half the population will be taking a drug of some kind. A survey of 9,000 Britons concluded that one in three people suffers from a long-standing illness or disability. Other surveys have shown that in any one 14 day period, 95% of the population consider themselves to be unwell for at least a few of those days. At no time in history has illness been so commonplace. We spend more than ever on health care but no one could argue that there is any less suffering in our society.

It is now widely accepted that at least 40% of all the people who are given prescription medicines will suffer uncomfortable, hazardous or potentially lethal side effects. And yet the vast majority of doctors never admit that their patients suffer any side effects. In Britain, for example, five out of six doctors have never reported any drug side effects to the authorities - authorities who admit that they receive information on no more than 10% - 15% of even the most serious adverse drug reactions occurring in patients. In other words they admit that they never hear about at least 85% - 90% of all dangerous drug reactions. Astonishingly, it is even accepted that some doctors will withhold reports of serious adverse reactions, and keep their suspicions to themselves, in the hope that they may later be able to win fame by publishing their findings in a journal or revealing their discovery to a newspaper or magazine.

Patients who take drugs are taking a risk; they are often taking part in a massive experiment and by taking a medicine may become worse off than if they had done nothing. To make things worse no one knows exactly how big the risks are when a particular drug is taken. All drugs are potential poisons that may heal or may kill.

The medical profession, the drug industry and the regulatory bodies all accept that the hazards of using any drug will only be known when the drug has been given to large numbers of patients for a considerable period of time. But no one seems particularly keen to monitor drugs which are being used. There is a vast and breathtaking shortage of common sense within the medical profession.

In October 2008, it was finally admitted that taking aspirin to prevent heart attacks might do more harm than good. Prior to that date many doctors were recommending that healthy patients took daily aspirin as a prophylactic. But I don't believe there was any convincing evidence showing that taking daily aspirin was safe. I had been so alarmed by the early research that I warned the instant it was published that the evidence didn't prove taking aspirin routinely was either safe or effective. My advice was ignored and sneered at but you have to ask yourself who benefitted most from the suggestion that vast numbers of healthy people should take a daily drug? Sir Richard Doll, who did some research on this issue, was, like many members of the medical establishment, later discredited. After his death it was revealed that he, like so many other eminent doctors, had received consultancy payments from chemical companies whose products he had defended. For example, he received $1,500 a day from Monsanto and had a `relationship' with the controversial company from 1976 until 2002.

In August 2010, the Government told doctors in Britain to weigh patients before giving them heparin. I have been screaming for years that this should be done for all drugs. It is utterly absurd that a seven stone woman should be given the same dose of a painkiller or antibiotic as a twenty stone man just because they are both `adults'. Why does it take doctors take so long to come to such obvious conclusions? The medical establishment lost touch with common sense a long, long time ago.

15. If You Want Holistic Medicine You Must Do It Yourself

There is a lot of talk about holistic medicine but there isn't much holistic medicine practised today. An intuitive, holistic approach goes against everything with which the bureaucratic, legalistic, constrained medical establishment feels comfortable. The medical establishment was bought by the drug industry decades ago. Modern medicine is geared to solving problems with drugs, surgery or radiotherapy and does not acknowledge the influence of stress or diet. Nor does the medical establishment appreciate the importance of preventive medicine. Doctors pay lip service to holistic medicine but what they really mean is that patients should be prepared to try a wide variety of drugs and orthodox medical treatments. Hospital specialists have drifted into intellectual parochialism. Most now specialise and then specialise again. They are absurdly narrow-minded and bigoted; there is no integration, no overview and no common sense.

Real holistic medicine means treating the patient in whatever way will produce effective, safe results. It means combining orthodox and alternative medicine. But whatever they may claim there are virtually no `holistic' hospitals in Britain. And there are no holistic healers. If you want holistic medicine then you must become a holistic patient. That's a tragedy because most patients don't have the knowledge or the confidence to do this.

`Holistic' (or, as it sometimes spelt, wholistic) medicine has, for several decades, been growing in theoretical popularity. Many alternative and some orthodox health care professionals describe themselves as `holistic' practitioners. But most aren't.

Most journalists inaccurately assume that the word is a synonym for `alternative' or `complementary' medicine.

But it isn't.

The word `holistic' was first introduced in 1926 by the South African philosopher and statesman Jan Christian Smuts. He suggested that the whole human being is much more than (and quite different to) a collection of physical or emotional parts. Even in those days, it seems, there must have been doctors parading up and down hospital wards referring to the `liver' in the end bed and the `case of pancreatitis' in the third bed on the left.

The word and the concept lay more or less forgotten until the 1970s when the growth of high technology medicine led to a revolution among patients who felt that aggressive, interventionist medicine wasn't entirely satisfactory. Suddenly there was a feeling that specialisation and fragmentation were not all they had been cracked up to be.

In practical terms the use of the word `holistic' meant, in theory at least, that instead of regarding patients as sick kidneys or hearts health care professionals would try to meet the physical, mental, emotional and spiritual needs of their patients by dealing with social problems as well as physical ones and by using natural healing methods as well as modern, pharmacological or surgical techniques.

In short, the word `holistic' was intended to describe an attitude. An attitude which can be just as well followed by an orthodox trained doctor as by an alternative practitioner. A general practitioner in a busy city health centre can be `holistic' in his approach just as easily as can a herbalist or acupuncturist working from a back bedroom.

There is no doubt that a truly `holistic' approach to medical care is extremely good news for patients. When followed properly it means that every illness can be treated with a `pick and mix' approach - choosing whichever aspects of orthodox and alternative medicine are most likely to be effective, and least likely to produce side effects, and treating and taking full notice of all aspects of the individual's being.

In many illnesses there is no point in treating what is wrong with the body unless you also treat what is wrong with the mind and it seems to me remarkable that a modern doctor will treat the body of a patient who is suffering from high blood pressure, irritable bowel syndrome or asthma but ignore the mind, when it is now established beyond doubt that in so many illnesses the physical symptoms are produced by mental turmoil of one sort or another. It is equally bizarre and, in truth, unscientific, for an osteopath to treat a patient's back and ignore his mind.

The advantages of a truly `holistic' approach are colossal not only because `holistic' medicine offers a chance to use the best and avoid the worst but also because different types of treatment can, when used together, have a synergistic effect. A genuinely `holistic' approach may use a modern drug, a relaxation technique and a type of massage to tackle a single collection of symptoms.

But although in theory the word `holistic' implies an admirable change in attitude there is, sadly, little evidence that practitioners really understand what the word means or how it should be applied in practice.

It would be nice to think that everyone could find a `holistic' practitioner to look after them. But don't hold your breath. You've about as much chance of striking oil when digging in your winter vegetables.

The myth that drug therapy offers the only true solution is now repeated unquestioningly and without hesitation or embarrassment. Many members of the medical establishment believe that medical advances largely depend upon the pharmaceutical industry. This is not regarded as a subject for debate but as a fundamental building block; a fact of medical life.

It is not surprising, therefore, that the drug company owned and controlled medical establishment still looks with horror at all varieties of alternative medicine. Attempts to organise research programmes into the effectiveness of acupuncture, herbalism or homoeopathy are invariably treated with a sneer or a patronising dismissal.

It is one of the great scandals of the 21st century that the billion dollar worldwide cancer industry, the international drug industry and the medical `profession' (now, more of a trade than a `profession') would all much rather suppress an alternative cancer treatment rather than have to admit that orthodox remedies might be bettered.

I don't think that many patients are ever going to receive truly `holistic' treatment from their practitioners. Most training programmes are, by their very nature, designed to produce specialists. Medical schools turn out drug dispensers and cutters. And there aren't many health care professionals with the time or inclination to study other available specialities.

We must also recognise that there is, of course, a huge financial disincentive involved here. How many practitioners are going to suggest to a paying patient that he would obtain better treatment by visiting another professional?

All this is sad.

But it doesn't mean that `holistic' medicine is out of reach. What it does mean is that if you really want `holistic' treatment (and in my opinion you should) you're going to have to take control yourself if you or anyone in your family needs treatment.

16. The NHS Has Too Much Money (But Wastes Most Of It)

It is constantly claimed that the NHS needs more money. This is a lie of political proportions. The people who work for it (and who have their snouts deep in the trough) are forever claiming that the organisation is underfunded. They are, of course, lying. And their lies are inspired by self-interest.

Throwing money at the NHS won't solve any of its problems. The sick joke is that the NHS already has too much money. What it lacks is leadership. No one in charge seems to know how money and resources should be spent. Employees spend most of their working hours finding new ways to grab as much of it as they can for themselves. They spend the rest of their time avoiding responsibility (legal and moral) and work. Patients wait for hours in casualty departments and for months for life saving surgery because money is wasted on pot plants, fancy furniture and obscene salaries for regiments of besuited men and women who contribute nought point zilch to patient care.

One basic problem with the NHS is that the people who work for it aren't spending their own money. And when people aren't spending their own money they do reckless, thoughtless things. The staff waste and steal.

I know of so many ways in which money is wasted or stolen by NHS employees that I hardly know where to begin. Hospital consultants who have private patients as well as NHS responsibilities often arrive hours late or slip away a few hours early - leaving their NHS patients to be looked after by young doctors who are supposed to be being trained. Consultants who do this are stealing time - and money - from the NHS. Bureaucrats, nurses and orderlies steal food, toilet rolls, disinfectant, writing paper, pens, envelopes and so on. Doctors tend to be more ambitious. They steal expensive bits of equipment which they use to equip their private consulting rooms. The amount of money wasted because employees fail to turn off lights that aren't needed - or to turn down heating that isn't necessary - would pay for the building and running of several new hospitals. Millions more are wasted on pointless and stupid paperwork and bureaucracy. The NHS must surely be the most bureaucratic and inefficient organisation in Britain. Vast amounts of money are wasted on handing out redundancy payments to NHS employees who have a weekend off and then find themselves being rehired - either as full time NHS staff or as private consultants. The greed of the Government in pushing the price of a prescription up beyond the price of many constituent drugs has made life very easy for thieves. The patient hands over a prescription and the required bundle of cash (one prescription charge for every item on the form). If the drug being prescribed is available without a prescription - and costs less than the prescription charge - the pharmacist simply tosses the prescription into the bin and keeps the price difference.

Not even privatising NHS hospitals has eradicated the waste. There are some former NHS hospitals which are now run as purely private hospitals and there is some irony in that it was a Labour Government which put dozens of NHS hospitals into private hands through its absurd `Private Finance Initiative'. Privatisation of health services through the Private Finance Initiative might have sounded a good idea to someone but the NHS now pays a fortune for having some of its hospital run for it. For example, one PFI contractor was recently revealed to have charged the NHS Ł333 to change a single light fitting in a hospital. (There are no decimal points missing, the sum charged really was Ł333.) That contractor subsequently made a profit of Ł37 million pounds when it sold its stake in the management of a former NHS hospital to a bank. Just how the nation benefitted from this piece of accounting nonsense I cannot imagine.

In October 2010, there was much fuss about the fact that Monaco resident and frock salesman Sir Philip Green had, after an investigation, discovered that civil servants waste lots of money when buying office paper and other essentials. I can guarantee that nothing much will happen. In the early 1980s I exposed NHS waste in some articles in the *Daily Star* (where I was a columnist at the time). I wrote the exposé after I received a computer print-out from a reader showing that the NHS was paying more for staples such as pens, paper and toilet rolls than I would pay if I bought them one at a time at a local supermarket. The editor told me that the Prime Minister was much excited by this and gave copies to every cabinet member. There was a great flurry of activity in Whitehall in general and in the NHS in particular but, of course, whenever anything is exposed any official department's first response is to search for the leak, rather than deal with the problem and so the NHS initiated an immediate enquiry designed not to find out why billions were being wasted but to discover how I had found out that billions were being wasted. The inquiry didn't find out anything which wasn't entirely surprising because (apart from the person who had given it to me) there was only one person in the world who knew where I'd acquired my information and they didn't bother to ask me. (I wouldn't have told them anything if they had bothered to ask me but they didn't know that.)

And yet whenever taxes rise the Government claims the extra money is needed for the NHS.

But money won't cure what's wrong with the NHS.

The principle problem is that the NHS has become a bureaucratic monster. There are now more administrators than hospital beds in the NHS. The damned administrators are probably even more numerous than the cockroaches - and considerably less useful. (The cockroaches do at least clear up bits of food left rotting on the floor).

And it isn't just administrators. The NHS is also heavily laden with committees, advisors and quangos. There are thousands of them. The bill for their tea and biscuits alone would pay for a few thousand more nurses. Any business which tried to cope with the input from so many amateurs would be a disaster. The solution is to share the authority out among the people who have the responsibility. And that is never going to happen within the NHS.

17. When Trials Are Tribulations

One of the major reasons for the disastrously high incidence of problems associated with drug use is the fact that the initial clinical trials, performed before a drug is made available for all general practitioners to prescribe for their patients, rarely involve more than a few thousand patients. Some initial trials may involve no more than half a dozen patients.

However, it is now well-known that severe problems often do not appear either until at least 50,000 patients have taken a drug or until patients have used a drug for many months or even years. Because of this a huge death toll can build up over the years. Drug control authorities admit that when a new drug is launched no one really knows what will happen or what side effects will be identified.

Doctors and drug companies are, it seems, using the public in a constant, ongoing, mass testing programme. And the frightening truth is that far more people are killed as a result of prescription drugs (including vaccines) than are killed as a result of using illegal drugs such as heroin or cocaine.

Doctors remain committed to the inadequate, preliminary trials because they get paid to perform them. In America, doctors who do trials for drug companies can earn an extra Ł650,000 a year. One company paid doctors Ł27,300 for every patient used in a trial. Academics are paid grants to work as consultants for drug companies. They receive fat fees for writing and speaking. They are given shares and royalties and they are allowed to put their names on articles written by company staff. A survey showed that a third of medical articles published are written by authors who hold a patent related to the invention they were writing about, or who were employees or shareholders in the company exploiting the research or were members of a board of advisors to a drug company or held some other financial interest. None of the papers published mentioned the authors' financial interests.

NHS patients are frequently used in clinical trials, without regard for their own symptoms or needs. Patients are given drugs that need testing. Doctors, torn between loyalty to their patients and loyalty to the drug companies, tend to swing easily in one direction and the result is that patients who have a low or non-existent chance of benefitting from a trial are put at risk simply so that drug companies and doctors can make money. Patients in stage 1 trials are unlikely to gain anything. They believe that their doctor is trying out a wonderful new drug on them but in reality they are doing toxicity tests - which may be very dangerous. Their doctor, however, will make a big chunk of money.

Another problem is that research produced by drug companies is provably biased. One critic recently assessed the published studies where one non-steroidal anti-inflammatory drug had been compared to another. He concluded:`In every single trial, the sponsoring company's drug was either equivalent to or better than, the drug is was compared to: all the drugs were better than all the other drugs.'

On top of all this, drug companies sometimes refuse to allow publication of articles which are critical about their drugs. Articles which draw attention to problems are suppressed. Doctors who want their articles published learn to say good things when they write about pharmaceutical products.

18. If You Are Over 50 Your Government Wants You Dead

In Britain, it is now official Government policy to ignore the needs of the elderly. Doctors and nurses are told to let old people die - and to withhold treatment which might save their lives. Hospital staff are told to deprive the elderly of food and water so that they die rather than take up hospital beds. Nursing home staff have even been given the right to sedate elderly patients without their knowledge. The only -ism that no one cares about is ageism.

But at what age are patients simply allowed to die? And how old is too old for patients to be resuscitated? At what point does society have the right to say `You've lived long enough, now you must die and make way for someone else'? And why should resuscitation be decided by age? It is possible to argue that it would make as much sense to decide according to wealth or beauty. But ageism is now officially accepted. Anyone over 60 is now officially old, though in a growing number of hospitals the cut off age for resuscitation is 55.

We live in a politically correct world but the elderly don't count - particularly if they are white and English. Report after report after report shows elderly patients being left in pain, in soiled bed clothes.

Elderly patients in hospital are ignored by staff and left to starve to death, denied even water if they cannot get out of bed and fetch it themselves.

Old people are a burden which the Government cannot afford and so the politicians will continue to authorise whatever methods are necessary to ensure that the number of burdensome old people is kept to a minimum. The existence of an absurd branch of medicine called geriatrics is used as an excuse to shove old people into backwater wards and to provide them with second-rate medical treatment. In February 2011, an official report condemned the NHS for its `inhumane treatment of elderly patients' and stated that NHS hospitals were `failing to meet even the most basic standards of care' for the over-65s. It is no exaggeration to say that the NHS treats the elderly with contempt. (It used to be said that you can judge a civilisation by the way it treats its elderly.)

It was back in February 2005 that it was revealed that the Government had advised that hospital patients with little hope of recovery should be allowed to die because of the cost of keeping them alive. The Labour Government suggested that `old people' be denied the right to food and water if they fell into a coma or couldn't speak for themselves. So much for any hope for stroke victims. The Government suggested that the need to cut costs came before the need to preserve the lives of patients and decided it had the right to overturn a right-to-life ruling which had been made when a judge ordered that artificial nutrition and hydration should not be withdrawn unless the life of a patient could be described as `intolerable'. (The judge had added that when there was any doubt, preservation of life should take precedence.)

Of course, depriving the elderly of food and water is sometimes more a consequence of incompetence than official policy. When my mother was in hospital in Exeter she couldn't feed herself but the staff didn't feed her. If no relative could get to the hospital to feed her she didn't eat. Drinks were put on her tray and then taken away untouched. `Not thirsty, today?' an idiot would ask merrily.

Meanwhile, the Government pours money into subsidising the lives of the lazy and the work-shy. Healthy 30-year-olds sit around growing chip backsides and beer bellies, slumped in front of their high definition digital television sets watching their choice of State subsidised satellite television, opening the windows to let the heat out because it's easier than turning down the central heating.

The elderly are classified as the `Unwanted Generation': a political embarrassment. Elderly individuals facing blindness from age-related macular disease are denied drugs that might have prevented their blindness. The elderly are considered expensive, useless and expendable. The theory is that they don't contribute and rarely vote and can, therefore, be disregarded. But those who believe this will be old sooner than they think. And the definition of 'old' is getting younger by the year.

Wars have taught us that people seem to be prepared to accept as normal all sorts of terrible things. But how unbelievably awful it is that doctors and nurses accept that the elderly (officially the over 60s) must be allowed to die because keeping them alive isn't cost effective. The official attitude seems to be that old people don't matter and don't have rights simply because they are old. In mid August 2007, a Select Committee on Human Rights, comprised of MPs and peers, reported that 21% of hospitals and care homes failed to meet even minimum standards of dignity and privacy for older people. The Committee said it had uncovered evidence of neglect, abuse, discrimination and unfair treatment of frail, older people. (Their discovery came as no surprise to those of us who have been uncovering such abuse for decades.) How have we managed to forget that in the 1930s the Nazis deliberately starved and dehydrated elderly and vulnerable patients because they were regarded as a useless burden on society? That is exactly what we are doing today.

An astonishing (and horrifying) survey conducted among readers of the journals *Nursing Standard* and *Nursing Older People* showed that fewer than one in six nurses said that nothing would prevent them from reporting abuse of older people in their care.

In other words five out of six nurses would, at least sometimes, fail to report abuse of the elderly people they were being paid to look after. So, in my view, five out of six of nurses aren't fit to be nurses.

Would these same nurses ignore the abuse of children so easily?

I suspect not.

This is utterly appalling and an indictment of the modern nursing profession.

The same survey showed that six out of ten nurses would turn a blind eye to the abuse of the elderly. They would say nothing if they knew that an elderly patient or care home resident was being beaten, bullied or robbed.

Why are nurses failing their patients?

One reason is cowardice.

Unbelievably, it seems that nurses are frightened to report abuse in case they themselves are abused by the person doing the abuse.

Oh, please.

Another reason is, apparently, `fear of misinterpreting the situation'.

What sort of political correct garbage is that?

Hospital patients and nursing home residents now often suffer malnutrition and dehydration, abuse and rough treatment, lack of privacy, neglect, poor hygiene and bullying. Thousands and thousands of elderly people are left for hours in soiled clothes.

How can anyone `misinterpret' any of that?

And *why?*

I'll tell you why.

Can it be because too many modern nurses are lazy, stupid and incompetent. Too many are far too self-important to do anything other than stare at a computer screen all day long.

In my view, nurses who say nothing when they see abuse are as guilty as the abusers. A once great profession is, today, in a worse state than it was in the days of Dickens. Is it so very old-fashioned of me to believe that every nurse should always report every incident of abuse? Always. Without exception.

Ageism is, it seems, now endemic in health care. A reader wrote to tell me that when she visited her doctor complaining of painful knees her doctor told her, very abruptly, that her problem was that she was living too long. She was devastated. `It wasn't said as a joke,' she told me. `He meant it.' In the months before he died my father repeatedly complained: `People treat me like a fool because I am old'. A 79-year-old reader told me: `If you are over 55 they want you dead because you're too expensive alive.'

We now live in a world where it is considered acceptable for men and women to have to share a ward; where hospital bathrooms are so dirty that patients dare not use them; where dentists are so scarce and expensive that people have to resort to pulling their own bad teeth with the aid of a length of string tied to a doorknob. But it is the elderly who, above all others, are regarded as disposable and irrelevant. It is the elderly who have no rights. Sexism and racism are outlawed but ageism is not. Indeed, it seems clear that ageism is now a State sponsored prejudice. Violent, feral youths who are caught assaulting elderly law-abiding citizens are likely to be 'punished' with a fistful of vouchers entitling them to a handful of free CDs (the lyrics of which may well encourage more violence) but honest, elderly citizens who, cannot afford to pay their council tax bill will end up in prison.

When doctors are owned by the Government then the Government's priorities take over. And so the elderly, who are regarded as an expensive burden, are considered expendable.

19. Your Doctor Will Kill You Now: The Cruel Waiting Game

Waiting lists are virtually unknown in other countries and they exist in Britain only because the NHS exists. If there were no NHS there would be no waiting lists. I have often found it difficult to explain the concept of a waiting list to see a doctor (let alone for essential life-saving surgery) to foreign doctors and patients.

The sad truth is that hardly anyone in the health care industry seems to give a damn about patients any more. As a doctor I have been embarrassed for years by the way patients are now treated. I have heard of patients kept waiting for hours in outpatient departments because 60 people were all booked in at 2.00 p.m. Weary, anxious patients then had two minutes with a junior doctor because the consultant who was paid to see them was seeing his private patients. Patients often think themselves lucky if the junior doctor who sees them speaks more than two words of English.

But keeping patients waiting isn't just a sign of rudeness on the part of the doctors. It can be deadly. And it now affects all areas of medical practice in Britain. Patients wait six months for vital X-rays. They wait weeks before they are told the results of laboratory tests. None of this is excusable. It happens because no one gives a damn. While patients and relatives suffer enormously the results they are waiting for sit on a desk, in a file or on a secretary's computer. Hospital staff either don't have any compassion or else they are determined sadists.

When I was a medical student and young doctor I remember being appalled to see obvious health problems in other countries. As I travelled around I spotted all sorts of untreated diseases: skin cancers, hernias, enlarged thyroids, dislocated hips and so on. It was difficult to travel through countries such as Turkey, Greece or North Africa without seeing a wide variety of untreated pathology. Now, in the UK, I often see people walking around with untreated pathology. They are, presumably, on someone's waiting list.

A reader wrote to tell me that she had been told by a doctor at the local hospital that she needed to have a barium enema examination to see if she had any serious bowel disease. `I assume that he is talking about cancer' she wrote. `But I have to wait 26 weeks before I can have the test done. Is it safe to wait that long?'

Of course it isn't safe to wait six months (or anything like that long) for a vital test which may show whether or not a cancer is developing. Some cancers can develop quickly and will, if left to develop unhindered for six months, become inoperable. By the time the barium enema result is available the patient could be dead.

Politicians (whose only specialist subjects are self-aggrandisement and self-enrichment) and media commentators (who do not understand very much about medical care) always give the impression that hospital waiting lists for surgery are all that really counts. This is nonsense. A patient who is ill and needs medical care can expect to have to have to wait not once but at least three times.

The first wait will be for the initial hospital outpatient appointment. It is not unknown for patients to have to wait a year for this preliminary appointment.

The second wait will be for the tests and investigations which the consultant considers necessary. A patient may have to wait another year for all these vital tests to be done. And then, when the tests have been done, there will be another wait for the results.

A reader of mine had a biopsy to find out whether or not a lump in her breast was cancerous. She had to wait three weeks before she received the result. (It was, inevitably, posted to her second class.) 'I nearly killed myself several times,' she told me. 'The pain of waiting was almost unbearable.'

When I was a young house surgeon I remember that it was not unusual for a surgeon to perform a breast biopsy on a patient on the operating table. The surgeon would then send the biopsy sample to the laboratory and have a cup of tea while he waited for the results. The anaethestist would keep the patient unconscious. If the biopsy showed a cancer then the surgeon would continue with whatever operation he felt necessary. (The patient would have signed a consent form before leaving the ward.) If the biopsy showed that the lump was benign the patient would be awoken, sent back to the ward and given the good news. So why does it now take three weeks to produce results which can be produced in minutes? Any doctor who doesn't provide a patient with such results on the same day is a psychopathic bastard.

Doctors and hospitals are often appallingly and inexcusably slow. I have on my desk a letter sent by a GP to his female patients inviting them for a smear test to see if they had cervical cancer. They would, he told them, expect to have the result of their test in 13 weeks. Thirteen weeks! The unnecessary worry caused by a delay of this length will, I suspect, mean that the smear testing activities of this doctor do far more harm than good.

I've also received a letter sent out telling women suspected of having breast cancer that they must expect to wait as much as 17 weeks for an NHS test. I wonder how many know that by the time they have the test (and the results) they may well be incurable. (This does nothing to damage NHS success rates. A patient is only officially recorded as suffering from cancer on the date when she is diagnosed. The 17 week wait isn't counted.)

In 2010, my wife was suspected of having motor neurone disease. Several weeks after the tests had been done we still had not received the results. It seemed difficult to understand why. When my wife telephoned the hospital to see if they had the results of her tests she spoke to a secretary who reported that the letter telling her whether or not she had motor neurone disease had yet to be typed. And when it had been typed it would still have to be signed. My wife asked if the letter could be faxed. She was told it could not. Exacerbated by the stress her symptoms became worse than ever. A few days later I telephoned the hospital. The registrar was off sick. I was told that the letter telling my wife whether or not she had motor neurone disease had been typed but that it was waiting to be signed. I told the secretary to whom I spoke that the inmates of Guantanamo are treated better. She said that the letter would be sent when ready. I then pointed out that we had been waiting nearly three weeks to find out whether or not my wife had a fatal disease. I also pointed out that we had not once met her consultant. I added that when we went for nerve conduction tests two other men (one of them not medically qualified) had been invited to view. I told the secretary that my wife had been extremely embarrassed when told to remove her tights in front of the three men. There was no screen and no nurse. I added that I have a medical degree, am a registered and licensed GP and am a Professor of Holistic Medical Sciences and finally I said that under all the circumstances it might be a good idea if they faxed the letter to us that afternoon. An hour or so later the fax machine purred into life and the fax came through. All the tests were negative. My wife did not have motor neurone disease. She refused to go back to the hospital ever again. She said she would rather just wait and see what happened.

In the end it turned out that the letter had been dictated on 21st July 2010. It was typed on 5th August 2010. It was finally posted on 17th August 2010 and it arrived on the 19th August 2010.

Later, my wife was sent an NHS appointment which she cancelled. The hospital told her that if she cancelled again they wouldn't let her have any more appointments. And they wanted to know why she was cancelling. (They had arbitrarily chosen the date and had given about one week's notice).   There's another problem.

Patients sometimes die untreated because doctors will not (or dare not) start any treatment until all the investigations have been completed. The fear of litigation means that doctors insist on waiting for written evidence before trying anything. Inevitably, this means that it is not infrequently too late to act by the time treatment is started. If, for example, there are two or three possible diagnoses available and only one of the diseases can be treated then it would seem to make sense to start the treatment for the disease which can be treated, even though laboratory evidence in support of that diagnosis might not be available. But this isn't what happens.

Finally, once the tests have been done, and the results obtained, the doctor will have to decide on the appropriate treatment: surgery, drugs or whatever else he considers most appropriate. At this stage it is, today, quite customary for NHS patients to have to wait 18 weeks before starting essential treatment. This is regarded as the target. This is not, of course, the sort of time that politicians or their families would be prepared to wait for treatment. And it is, remember, a target. In reality, many patients wait far longer than this.

It is the third type of wait, the wait for treatment, which makes up official hospital waiting lists. When politicians talk about there being a million patients awaiting treatment they are referring to this list - not to the other two lists.

The wait for treatment can be haunting and enormously stressful. Patients who need radiotherapy are supposed to receive it within four weeks but two thirds have to wait longer than that. Recent figures show that NHS patients with breast cancer wait up to 119 days for radiotherapy. If the radiotherapy is essential then they really might as well not bother. In fact the 119 days wait was the average at the hospitals managed by Oxford Radcliffe Hospitals NHS Trust, and patients referred for breast clinic assessments had to wait up to 126 days for their initial appointment so it seems fair to add the 126 days onto the 119 days. The reasons given were a shortage of equipment and of radiographers. I bet there were plenty of administrators.

Incidentally, when the 202 hospitals in England which give radiotherapy to breast cancer patients were asked to give information about their waiting times more than half (113) failed or refused to give any information so it is a fair bet many were much longer than 119 days.

(Just why do administrators think they have the right to keep such vital information secret?)

In my view any doctor who works at a hospital with outrageously long waiting times for cancer patients needing treatment should be struck off for unprofessional conduct. Someone really should be forced to take responsibility for something within the NHS. And the simple fact is that waiting lists are probably three times as bad as most people think they are - for the simple reason that patients have to wait three separate times for medical attention. And waiting is dangerous. It can kill you.

The idea of patients having to wait for essential, and possibly life-saving treatment, is something we've got used to. But Britain is the only country in the world where patients routinely have to wait for weeks, months or even years for essential treatment. Patients and doctors in other countries don't even understand the concept of a waiting list.

Waiting lists were originally an invention of part-time NHS consultants who wanted to boost their earnings from private patients. They kept their NHS lists long to encourage patients to pay for treatment. I first revealed this scandal in 1986. I was attacked rather viciously by many doctors at the time. But no one has bothered to deny the truth of this for a long time.

Today things are infinitely worse.

NHS hospitals have themselves become dependent on the extra income they receive from private patients. They need the cash desperate patients pay for investigations and treatment in order to pay the hugely inflated salary bill for administrators and managers.

Hospitals make money this way because even full-time salaried NHS hospital consultants (the ones who have signed contracts promising to work full-time for the NHS rather than to share their working lives between NHS and private patients) are now allowed to charge patients for private treatment - and to pocket the money they make. Since they don't have private consulting rooms, or private hospital facilities available, they are, of course, allowed to use NHS facilities, NHS equipment and NHS staff. They are even allowed to use NHS secretaries, NHS stationery and NHS stamps to deal with the paperwork (such as sending out appointments and bills).

NHS hospitals have always allowed some consultants to choose between working full-time for the NHS and working part-time. Those consultants who chose to work part-time were paid less but allowed to spend some of their working week seeing private patients. However, NHS hospitals now allow all NHS consultants (including those who are supposed to be working full time for the NHS) to charge extra fees for seeing private patients and the NHS has created (and is itself now addicted to) a two tier health system. Effectively, what happens is that NHS hospitals sell patients the chance to jump the waiting list. Patients see full time NHS consultants in NHS hospitals but if they pay everyone concerned a fee they don't have to wait in the normal NHS way.

As the NHS deteriorates so consultants are charging more for NHS appointments and, at the same time, reducing the length of time they allow for each consultation. Proper private patients (seen in private hospitals or consulting rooms) used to be seen for an hour - giving them time to talk, explain and ask questions. Patients seeing consultants privately in private consulting rooms may still be allowed this amount of time. But patients seeing consultants privately in NHS hospitals are lucky to spend ten or fifteen minutes with the consultant. That's about the sort of time they might hope to have devoted to them if they saw the consultant as NHS patients. The difference? The payment entitles them to jump the queue.

The private patient who sees a consultant in an NHS hospital will be treated just as badly as an NHS patient. There are no soft chairs, cups of tea and expensive magazines because they wait in the same NHS waiting room that NHS patients use. For this rudimentary service, patients, who are invariably frightened and reluctant to question the bills they are given, are charged extortionate prices.

Rude, uncaring consultants, operating from the security of NHS premises, and using NHS facilities (including NHS secretarial services) may charge Ł400 to Ł600 for a brusque and snarly service. Because patients are desperate not to have to wait six months to see a consultant, and because they have no way of knowing what is fair, prices have gone through the roof. I know of consultants who charge Ł500 to look at an X-ray and write a two line report.

A reader wrote to me recently to report that when she had a private appointment with an NHS consultant she was kept waiting 30 minutes in a crowded, noisy and, rather scruffy and untidy waiting room before being rushed into the consulting room for a hurried ten minute consultation. No one apologised for the fact that she was kept waiting 30 minutes for her appointment. `It reminded me,' she wrote, `of the NHS as it was a decade or two ago.' She is not alone in her observation. The truth is that the NHS has deteriorated to a level which would have been considered utterly unacceptable a decade ago, while private medicine, offering the only alternative and with standards largely set by NHS staff, has drifted downwards too.

This massive NHS fraud goes on (and is actively encouraged) because it isn't just the consultants (already paid to work full-time looking after NHS patients but cheating on their contracts by seeing patients privately while they are also being paid by the NHS) who make extra money. NHS hospitals can also boost their income by allowing patients who can afford to pay to jump the queues for tests or surgery. Administrators support this abuse of the system because their hospitals are so bloated with expensive bureaucrats that they need the private fees. While the full-time NHS consultant is allowed to cheat and charge a fee for the opportunity to jump the waiting queue, the hospital also charges the patient an extortionate fee for the privilege of using the NHS waiting room and other NHS hospital facilities. The present corrupt system is likely to continue for as long as everyone is making extra money. And, of course, as long as this corrupt system continues, doctors and hospitals will benefit from deliberately keeping their NHS waiting lists as long as possible. If the waiting lists aren't kept long there won't be any NHS patients prepared to pay hard cash for the chance to live. In the 21st century NHS, the rich may live but the poor will die.

Several hundred thousand people a year pay privately so that they can jump the NHS waiting list. Heaven knows how many more pay privately for X-rays and scans. It's impossible to say how much we are talking about but this is undoubtedly a multi-billion pound a year scam. If this were happening somewhere hot, dusty and far away, indignant MPs would be standing up wagging fingers and there would be programmes on our televisions about it.

The NHS now offers a two tier service. Money doesn't buy better care. But it buys faster care. And that's crucial.

The way this works in practice is alarmingly simple.

You go to your GP because you have stomach pains and are vomiting blood. You have lost a good deal of weight in a month. Dr Harold Shipman, your friendly GP, who is having a good day because the nurse has earned him another Ł5,000 by jabbing several hundred children with a lethal cocktail of some fashionable vaccine, gives you two minutes of his valuable time and decides that you need to have some tests done since you might have cancer of the stomach. Dr Shipman tells you that he will send you to see Dr Hans Kneesandbumpsadaisy in the outpatient clinic at the local hospital. But, sadly, there is a 17 week wait for an appointment. And once you have had that preliminary appointment there will be a 22 week wait for the X-rays which will help Dr Kneesandbumpsadaisy reach a diagnosis. Dr Shipman and you both know that by that time you will probably be dead. There is, however, an alternative. If you can afford it you can pay to see Dr Kneesandbumpsadaisy privately. You see him in exactly the same outpatients department, at exactly the same NHS hospital, that you would have seen him in if you'd been prepared to wait until you died. You sit with the NHS patients who haven't paid but who were referred many weeks ago and who have managed to hang on for their first consultation. You only have to wait a week because you've paid to jump the queue. Dr Kneesandbumpsadaisy, employed full-time by the NHS, tells you that you need an X-ray. There is, he says, a waiting list of another 22 weeks to have this done but if you have more money and are prepared to pay his friend Dr Ebeneezer Sodoff, the radiologist, for a private consultation, you will only have to wait a week for the X-rays you need. The X-rays will be done in the same NHS hospital and in the NHS X-ray department where you would have had to go to as an ordinary NHS patient. Once again you will sit alongside NHS patients who have been waiting for months but you will have fast-tracked yourself. You will receive a bill from Dr Kneesandbumpsadaisy and another bill from Dr Sodoff. You will also receive a hefty bill from Mr Sticky-Fingers, the hospital administrator, because although you saw both NHS doctors in NHS facilities and both used NHS equipment you paid to cheat the system and jump the queue. All the work is done on NHS property, using NHS equipment and in time already paid for by taxpayers. Hospitals and consultants are unashamedly flogging off places higher up the waiting list. If there wasn't a waiting list they wouldn't have anything to sell.

Is it simple fraud? Is it just theft?

Or are you just bribing the doctors and the hospital so that you can jump the queue?

One thing is certain: if the NHS wasn't a State-owned and run institution, everyone involved would be learning to pick up the soap with their toes.

NHS hospitals charge the same fees as private hospitals, though they provide a much more basic service. (The precise fees vary from hospital to hospital. Doctors and administrators know that patients are usually too anxious and frightened to shop around to find the `best buy', and too ignorant to know whether they are being ripped off.) Similarly, consultants working in NHS hospitals invariably charge the same massive fees as genuinely private consultants - but they don't bother with the smiles, the handshakes, the comforting words or the expensive suits. They know that they're not selling `special care'. They're flogging a chance to be seen this week instead of next year. They're selling a chance to be treated before it's too late. They're flogging a chance to stay alive. You don't have to tart things up when you're selling life itself. They don't bother with expensive magazines, cups of tea and smiling receptionists. Neither doctors nor hospitals pretend to be offering anything more than a chance to be seen more speedily. Greedy consultants are getting rich, preying on patients who are struggling to stay alive in the wreckage of the NHS.

One reader of mine paid Ł200 to a full time NHS consultant for a standard 5 minute consultation in an NHS hospital. She had to pay the NHS hospital another Ł60 for the use of their grubby facilities. What did she get for her Ł260? Simply the chance to jump the queue.

Another reader had to pay Ł380 to a consultant who reported on a scan. The consultant hadn't even been there when the scan was done.

Most patients don't even ask how much the bill is going to be.

`If patients don't ask I don't tell them,' boasted one consultant. `If they want to know how much the bill will be it's up to them to ask.'

The modern NHS consultant has the best of both worlds. He combines a stable income, an excellent pension, sick pay cover and all the other perks of civil servant status with the ability to earn a vast amount through his `private patients'.

He doesn't even have to go out and find the private patients. The NHS finds them for him.

Doctors have become as greedy and grasping as a bunch of Arthur Daleys. They snatch every penny they can from frightened and desperate patients and their frightened and desperate relatives. And for doctors and hospitals there is a bonus: NHS patients who are seen as 'private' patients cannot use the NHS complaints machinery. The patient may have been seen in an NHS building by a salaried NHS doctor using NHS equipment and dictating his report to an

NHS secretary using NHS notepaper but if the patient has agreed to hand over money to jump the queue the hospital won't accept any complaint about itself or a doctor. Patients who pay to jump the queue lose all their rights and safeguards.

When the money runs out the patients simply go back into the NHS system and waits for the next instalment of their treatment.

(And don't think you can use the system and refuse to pay. The modern NHS consultant is quite likely to have an account with a local debt collector. If you haven't handed over your `bribe' money quickly enough you could have the doctor's hired thugs banging on your door.)

If all this sounds too bad to be true you can check it out for yourself in minutes. Pick a speciality (any speciality). Ring your nearest large NHS hospital and ask to speak to a secretary working for a consultant in that speciality. Name an operation or an investigation and ask how long the waiting list is. Then ask how long you'd have to wait if you paid for private care. Hospital managers don't try to hide what is happening. They brazenly admit that they're flogging places on the waiting list.

If waiting lists were to disappear NHS hospitals (and NHS consultants) would lose this nice little earner. Many NHS hospitals would go bust and a lot of NHS consultants would have to sell the second BMW and the chalet in Switzerland.

The current system means that the NHS is appallingly unfair. There have always been inequalities. Some areas have better hospitals than others. It's called a `National' Health Service but if you have a rare disease then your chances of surviving have always depended on where you live. But the way the NHS is now run is clearly divisive and grossly unequal. The NHS was founded to ensure that everyone got equal care - regardless of wealth. That was the whole idea of it. But the modern NHS is flourishing by taking advantage of the fact that some patients can afford to pay (or will find the money by selling the car or remortgaging the house). In today's NHS this new way of doing things mean that if you're poor and cannot afford to `buy' a higher place on the waiting list, your chances of surviving your illness are dramatically reduced.

The result is that neither NHS administrators nor NHS consultants want to get rid of waiting lists. Indeed, they have a vested interest in maintaining them and keeping them as long as possible. Bureaucrats are making huge salaries out of the modern, two-tier NHS. And consultants are making a fortune out of their bribes. The NHS is hooked on waiting lists. Neither consultants nor administrators can give them up because they are a great source of income. Waiting lists could be permanently and easily eradicated if doctors and administrators wanted to get rid of them. But they don't.

Meanwhile, long waiting times mean that thousands of people need to take huge amounts of time off work. Many then become accustomed to watching daytime television. They realise they are just as well off financially if they stay at home. The NHS is, therefore, partly responsible for the sick note culture. The resultant costs to the nation are massive.

I have for years been screaming about the fact that NHS staff deliberately increase waiting times in order to increase their profits from private medicine. I have repeatedly explained this to journalists but they either fail to understand the significance of this or they are unwilling to rock the sinking boat.

Finally, I can't leave the subject of hospital waiting times without drawing attention to the fact that emergency patients now have to wait too.

Imagine: your child breaks an arm. You have to rush him to hospital. This is not a routine appointment for varicose veins. This is an emergency. Which is why you take him direct to the nearest Accident and Emergency Department. (Your local hospital may not have one of these and if you turn up at a hospital without an accident department you will be turned away and told to take him elsewhere.)

You expect, of course, that your child will be seen within minutes and that he will be treated straight away.

Wrong.

The officially acceptable wait for treatment in an Accident and Emergency department is four hours. The average wait is seven hours. Can you imagine the Prime Minister standing waiting for seven hours before his child is attended to?

The Government has run an expensive campaign telling the relatives of stroke victims to ensure that they get to hospital quickly because urgent treatment can reduce the seriousness of a stroke. What's the point in hurrying when you are going to have a seven hour wait when you get there? Horror stories abound. A reader of mine, distressed, bleeding and in pain, had a miscarriage and had to wait nine hours in hospital before she was seen.

NHS staff complain that they get shouted at, abused and occasionally attacked. I'm not surprised. The only thing that surprises me is that there are some NHS staff members who aren't attacked. It is, to be honest, a surprise that every NHS staff member isn't walking on crutches. Only the English, self-effacing to the point of being self-destructive, would put up waiting seven hours for emergency medical treatment. And if people who used the NHS knew exactly what was going on there would be rioting in the streets.

Incidentally, waiting times in institutionalised accident and emergency departments are awful but it seems that the worst thing anyone can do is to drive a patient to hospital in an emergency. If you arrive in an ambulance you have a chance of being seen relatively quickly. If you arrive by private transport you could wait for hours longer - even if you are clutching an arm which has been severed and is wrapped in a wet cloth. You could, indeed, be placed on a trolley and simply forgotten. Until someone else needs the trolley and finds you there. Dead.

20. Doctors Get Their Timing Wrong

It has been known for centuries that the leaves of some plants regularly open during the daytime and close at night. It was always assumed that this phenomenon was a response to sunlight. But over two 250 years ago, in 1729, a French astronomer called Jean-Jacques de Mairan, conducted a very simple experiment which showed that this assumption was wrong. He discovered that this phenomenon occurs even if a plant is kept in the dark. The only possible explanation was that the plant opens and closes in response to some sort of 24 hour internal clock. That was the first experiment in chronobiology.

Since then chronobiology (the study of temporal patterns related to biological phenomena) has become an acknowledged science. It is now known that just about every living organism - from a nucleated single cell to a human being - follows a 24 hour or circadian rhythm. So, for example, your pulse rate and blood pressure are highest first thing in the morning (with the result that the incidence of heart attack and stroke is highest at that time of day). In the evening your pulse rate and blood pressure will naturally fall. Your body temperature rises during the day and falls at night. Your blood platelets - which help with blood clotting - are stickier in the morning than at any other time of day. You are, therefore, likely to have less trouble with bleeding if you nick yourself in the morning than if you nick yourself in the evening. Your tolerance for alcohol peaks at five o'clock in the afternoon. And finally, most babies are born - and most people die - between the hours of midnight and dawn.

Our bodies respond in a cyclical way because we have evolved on earth - and the amount of light and heat and the level of electromagnetic and gravitational forces on our planet all vary in a rhythmic way.

The important thing - still widely ignored by doctors and many alternative health care professionals - is that the abnormalities associated with disease also vary in a cyclical and circadian way.

Whether you are suffering from cancer, heart disease, arthritis or asthma your disease will change during the day and, consequently, whatever you do to tackle the disease should also be arranged according to a circadian rhythm. For example, during the day and the night your body's ability to absorb drugs will vary. When given at the right time of day a drug will have a powerful and positive effect on an illness. But when given at the wrong time of day a drug may prove toxic.

Next, consider allergy reactions.

Allergy reactions develop when the body's natural defenses against foreign organisms over-react. If you are exposed to a pollen, or a type of food to which you are allergic, your body will send white blood cells to the site at which the foreign organisms have been spotted. The white cells will then proceed to eat up the foreign organisms. Some of the white cells release a substance called histamine which increases local blood flow and triggers the release of more white cells. The symptoms produced by this reaction include pain, itchiness, burning, redness and swelling.

Your body's ability to deal with outside threats in this way is influenced by the amount of glucocorticoid (a steroid hormone) in your blood stream. When the amount of glucocorticoid is at its highest your body's ability to deal with an outside organism will be at its lowest.

Now, under your body's circadian rhythm the amount of glucocorticoid in your blood is at its highest level in the morning - at around 5.00 a.m. or 6.00 a.m. Inevitably, therefore, your body's ability to deal with an external threat is lowest at this time of day.

But in the evening when your body's levels of glucocorticoid fall your body's ability to deal with a threat rises.

This means that you are least likely to develop an allergy reaction early in the morning. But, at that same time of day, you are also, because of the same effect, most susceptible to infection.

On the other hand you are most likely to develop an allergy reaction - and least susceptible to infection - in the evening.

(The fact that the body's levels of steroids are naturally highest early in the morning mean that a patient who has to take a steroid drug - which carries with it a risk of serious side effects - will probably suffer fewer side effects if he or she takes the drug very early in the day when the body is best prepared for it.)

Next, consider arthritis - a common inflammatory disease which also runs on a biological clock.

In rheumatoid arthritis the joints are attacked by a malfunctioning immune system. The joints of a rheumatoid arthritis sufferer are usually stiffest and most swollen early in the morning. They become easier during the day. In other types of arthritis - such as osteoarthritis - the stiffness and pain get worse during the day.

It is clear from this knowledge that the time when medication is given for these two different types of disease is vital. A drug given for rheumatoid arthritis should be timed to act in the morning, whereas a drug given for osteoarthritis should be timed to be working most efficiently later in the day.

Asthma is one of the commonest diseases in the world. It is getting commoner. (Although as I have explained in my book *How To Stop Your Doctor Killing You* I believe that many of the diagnoses of asthma - and other disorders - currently being made are false.) Because of the circadian rhythms associated with a number of normal physiological processes (such as airway size and breathing patterns) the majority of asthma attacks take place between 2.00 a.m. and 6.00 a.m. in the morning. The airways are naturally open widest during the day and there is a reduction in airflow after midnight.

Heart disease is linked to body rhythms (heart attacks are twice as common in the morning as they are during the rest of the day - making high stress breakfast meetings a risky venture).

The activity of cancer cells is also linked to body rhythms. Drugs prescribed to attack cancer usually operate by killing cells when they are most vulnerable - during the process of division. Anti-cancer drugs target cancer cells because cancer cells grow and divide far faster than other human body cells. However, other rapidly dividing cells (particularly cells inside the intestine and cells in the bone marrow) are likely to be killed unnecessarily by anti-cancer drugs. However, if an anti-cancer drug is given at the right time of day the problems associated with such a drug can be minimised and the effectiveness of the drug can be maximised. One trial showed that women with ovarian cancer who were given their drugs at the right time of day were four times as likely to survive for five years as other women - whose drug taking was not regulated in this way. Other researchers have found a similar difference when treating patients with colon cancer.

It isn't just drug therapy which is influenced by time. There is evidence which suggests that far more pre-menopausal women survive breast surgery if they have an operation which is done during the second half of their menstrual cycle than if they have an operation in the first two weeks of their cycle. This difference can probably be explained by the change in hormone levels which occurs during a menstrual cycle.   If researchers put more effort into studies of this sort, and wasted less time and money on pointless research such as animal experimentation, far more lives would be saved. The link between surgery, breast cancer, survival rates and the menstrual cycle was first observed in 1836 (yes, 1836 - over 175 years ago) so I really don't understand why more research hasn't been done to find out the precise link between hormone levels and cancer. If I were a woman having breast surgery for cancer I would *want* to have the operation done in the second half of my menstrual cycle (though I probably wouldn't be given the choice).

Any patient who needs drug therapy should ask their doctor to check if there is any evidence to show whether the treatment works best at a particular time of day. My guess is that most doctors will have never heard of chronobiology. But getting the timing right could make a life or death difference so it is well worth while being persistent.

This really is an area where more research is needed - and needed fast. It seems to me to be quite absurd that we have failed to pay much attention at all to this absolutely vital branch of medical science. Many deaths and a good deal of illness could be avoided by the expenditure of a relatively small amount of effort in this area. I don't have any doubt that timing is vital - for patients as well as for comedians. But, amazingly, it is a phenomenon that doctors still ignore - either simply because it's inconvenient and they're too lazy to bother with it, or because it isn't something that has yet been introduced into the official, established way of doing things.

21. The NHS Is Not Free

Consumers make the foolish, eternal mistake of assuming that, because no money changes hands at the point of sale, the NHS is `free'. It is a myth that the NHS is free. It is not free in any sense. It is extraordinarily expensive to run (far, far more expensive than an equivalent private health service would cost) and it is directly controlled by lobbyists and the politically motivated. Moreover, the financial cost is soaring. In 1996 the total bill for the NHS was Ł40,000,000,000. By 2010 the NHS was costing Ł104,000,000,000 a year to run. And, while health care costs are rising faster than just about any other costs, the quality of care provided by the NHS is falling at an unprecedented rate.

The cost of the NHS is rising because of the unbridled greed of doctors, nurses and drug companies, an absurd rise in the number of administrators required to design forms, hand them out, collect them and feed the results into computers and the continued incompetence of the people supposedly looking after the money. The NHS now costs so much that it would be cheaper to give every individual in the country free private medical insurance. The NHS costs around Ł1,750 a year for every man, woman and child. Have you had Ł1,750 worth of care out of the NHS this year? If everyone were given their Ł1,750 with which to buy private medical insurance each individual would have enough money left over to have an excellent annual holiday as well. And all the damned administrators, the leeches who have sucked the blood and the soul out of the NHS, would be released to find gainful employment. There must be something useful at least some of them could do.

Most of the extra money given to the NHS is spent on hiring more administrators, or giving pay rises to existing NHS staff. Patients don't benefit at all. Extra layers of administration mean that costs are constantly rocketing, while the quality of care steadily but remorselessly deteriorates. The NHS employs nearly 1.5 million people and more than 60% of those are bureaucrats. In addition to a Ministry, the health service is run by over 750 boards, committees, executive councils, local health authorities and quangos. Administration within the NHS is a sick joke. It's hardly surprising that doctors and nurses are demoralised and that patients are treated as a nuisance. Like other huge State industries the NHS has forgotten that it exists to serve. The system now has a bureaucratic life of its own and it sometimes seems as though senior NHS staff spend most of their time searching for new ways to waste money. For example, the NHS employs an army of translators in order to assist the many EU immigrants who haven't bothered to learn our national language.

Everything which the NHS publishes appears in a 160 languages. The cost of all this nonsense is one of the reasons why the NHS provides such appalling health care and such very poor value for money. For example, taken at random, I see that according to the latest available WHO figures, Singapore spends 3.4% of its GDP on health care (compared to 8.4% in the UK). And yet the infant mortality rate in Singapore is three per 1,000 whereas in the UK it is five per 1,000. And life expectancy at birth is higher in Singapore than in the UK. The WHO puts the UK in 18th place for health care provision. And that is truly appalling. It's no wonder that many immigrants (including illegal ones) pop back home if they fall ill and need medical treatment.

It is perhaps hardly surprising that no other country in the world has ever bothered to try to copy the British health care system. The NHS is so damned big that it can't do anything efficiently. Medical records take days to travel yards from one department to another and are regularly mislaid. Some time after my father died his missing hospital records were found in a wardrobe in a nursing home 20 miles away.

Senior doctors are silent about everything that goes on within the NHS because they have been bought. Hospital consultants who know the right people can receive an annual bonus which more or less doubles their standard NHS salary. A bonus of Ł70,000 or Ł80,000 is not unusual. These bonuses are awarded secretly and have nothing to do with patient satisfaction or reliable, honourable service to the NHS.

There is no doubt that one of the fundamental problems within the NHS is the cost of the workforce. Like almost all public sector workers they are overpaid and underworked. In Britain the average full time public sector employee works just 30 hours a week and much of that time is wasted on chatting, drinking coffee and filling in pointless forms. Within the NHS the figure is even worse because the size of the organisation, and the extent of the bureaucracy, mean that even when employees are doing what they regard as work they often are not doing anything useful. Employees in the private sector have to work much harder because any private hospital which tried to operate in the way that NHS hospitals operate would soon go bankrupt.

NHS hospitals are so out of touch with the needs of patients, and run by such uncaring, greedy people, that they now charge patients and visitors to park their cars. And since patients have no choice but to pay, the charges are extortionate. It is not unusual to find an NHS hospital charging Ł3 an hour. That's Ł9 for three hours, Ł12 for four hours and Ł15 if you're really ill and need to be there for five hours. These are prices that would make airport car park operators blush. And yet I have never seen a private hospital which charges patients or visitors to park their cars. The result is that sick people in the outpatients department sit and worry that they will be fined or clamped when they are kept waiting for hours. A recent survey showed that one quarter of people are put off visiting a friend or relative in hospital because of car park charges. Don't the malicious, mean-spirited, blood-sucking bastards who run our hospitals realise that visitors help patients get better?

Hospitals in the NHS are all about money. And the doctors and nurses who say nothing and allow the bureaucrats to get away with this obscene thugging of the sick are as guilty as the administrators themselves.

Finally, the NHS (like the rest of the State system) is designed to punish the prudent - especially the elderly prudent. Sick, elderly people are forced to sell their homes and use the proceeds to pay for essential care - even though, according to the law, the NHS should be picking up the bill. The NHS spends huge amounts of money evading this legal responsibility.

22. Bugs, Bugs, Glorious Bugs

A few decades ago the development of antibiotics led many people to believe that the threat offered by infectious diseases had, to a large extent, been conquered.

But a combination of greed and stupidity has changed all that. The effectiveness of antibiotics has been dramatically weakened by three main groups: the companies making them, the medical profession and the farming industry. Each of these groups has acted irresponsibly and dangerously. Since they cannot possibly have been unaware of the impact their actions would have, it is impossible to avoid the conclusion that the effectiveness of antibiotics has been deliberately destroyed for short-term profit. The drug companies, the medical establishment and the farming industry will together be responsible for millions of deaths around the world. The politicians who have stood to one side and allowed all this to happen must share the responsibility.

During the last few decades simple, widespread infections have been striking back and re-establishing themselves as serious threats to our health. Today, our hospitals are dangerous places for the healthy - and far too dangerous for the sick.

In 1952 virtually all infections caused by staphylococcus could be cured by penicillin. But just 30 years later a worrying 90% of patients infected with the staphylococcus bug needed treatment with other antibiotics. Western doctors didn't worry about this because they had other antibiotics to prescribe. With remarkable arrogance the medical profession in America and Europe assumed that it could always stay one step ahead of the bugs. What many doctors failed to realise was that yeasts, fungi and bacteria have been producing antibiotics more or less since time began. They use the antibiotics they make to protect themselves. Other yeasts, fungi and bacteria mutate naturally in order to protect themselves against those antibiotics. Through a mixture of ignorance and arrogance doctors speeded up the rate at which bugs acquired resistance, by spreading antibiotics around with reckless abandon. Overwhelmed by reckless enthusiasm, doctors started routinely giving antibiotics to all the patients whom they thought might be at risk - and this category often included all those patients who were destined for surgery. The prescribing doctors either didn't realise or didn't care that by dishing out antibiotics so freely they were giving the bacteria a greatly increased chance of acquiring immunity.

Staphylococcus has not, of course, been the only bug to become resistant and the Western medical establishment, constantly afraid of offending the drug companies, has done everything possible to stifle protests and warnings about the consequences. Today the future is truly bleak. Infectious diseases which we thought we had conquered are coming back with a vengeance. More and more people are dying of simple, uncomplicated infections. The bugs are getting stronger. And our ability to kill them is diminishing almost daily.

Today, one in six prescriptions is for an antibiotic and my educated guestimate is that between 50% and 90% of all these prescriptions are unnecessary or inappropriate. To a certain extent doctors over-prescribe because they like to do something when faced with a patient - and prescribing a drug is virtually the only thing most of them can do. And to some extent prescribing a drug is a defence against any possible future charge of negligence (on the basis that if the patient dies it is better to have done something than to have done nothing). But the main reason for the over-prescribing of antibiotics is, without doubt, the fact that doctors are under the influence of the drug companies. The makers of the antibiotics want their drugs prescribed in vast quantities. It makes no difference to them whether or not the prescriptions are necessary.

Things are made worse by the fact that although antibiotics have been around for over half a century, and the drug companies making them must have made billions of dollars in profits, no one yet knows how long antibiotic tablets should really be taken for when treating any specific condition. Should you take an antibiotic course for 5, 7, 10 or 14 days? The bizarre truth is that your guess is probably as good as your doctor's and his is probably as good as the drug company's.

The over-prescribing of antibiotics would not matter too much if these drugs were harmless and if there were no other hazards associated with their use. But antibiotics are certainly not harmless. The unnecessary and excessive use of antibiotics causes allergy reactions, side effects and a huge variety of serious complications - including the ultimate complication: death. And, of course, there is also the very real hazard that by overusing antibiotics doctors are enabling bacteria to develop immunity to these potentially life-saving drugs. There is now no doubt that many of our most useful drugs have been devalued by overuse and are no longer effective. The overprescribing of antibiotics is extraordinarily dangerous and constantly underestimated. It is far more of a threat to human life, and more of a threat to our future, than terrorism. The unnecessary antibiotics we have swallowed by the ton have weakened our general resistance to infection and paradoxically, strengthened the power of the bugs.

The existence of many antibiotic-resistant organisms is the main reason why infections are such a major problem in hospitals. Alarmingly, at least 1 in 20 of all hospital patients will pick up an infection in hospital - mostly urinary tract, chest or wound infections. The spread of these antibiotic-resistant organisms is mostly caused by doctors and nurses failing to wash their hands often enough. The problem is so great that the extra costs incurred when doctors have to prescribe increasingly expensive antibiotics are beginning to add an enormous burden to all those responsible for providing health care facilities. In America the extra cost of dealing with antibiotic-resistant organisms is many billions of dollars a year.

Partly thanks to doctors and drug companies the future is truly bleak. Infectious diseases which we thought we had conquered are coming back with a vengeance. More and more people are dying of simple, uncomplicated infections. The bugs are getting stronger. And our ability to kill them is diminishing almost daily.

However, the problem isn't entirely the result of overprescribing by doctors. The overuse of antibiotics by farmers is another big reason why infectious diseases are making a dramatic comeback. Astonishingly, considerably more than half of all the antibiotics sold are given by farmers to healthy animals.

Farmers claim that their animals are only given antibiotics when they have been recommended by a vet. Of course this is true. Farmers cannot buy antibiotics without a vet. But sadly, there are enough money hungry vets around to make sure that any farmer who wants to give his animals continuous doses of antibiotics will have no supply problem. I talked to one vet who regularly prescribed huge quantities of antibiotics for farmers to give to healthy cattle. `Don't you realise that what you are doing is endangering the lives of millions of human beings?' I asked him. He shrugged; he clearly knew I was right but clearly didn't care. `Why do you do it?' I asked him. `The farmers demand them,' he said with blunt honesty. `If I don't prescribe antibiotics someone else will and I'll lose the farm business.'

Why do farmers give their animals so many antibiotics?

Well, some, of course, are prescribed to help prevent (and treat) disease. Animals on modern western farms are exceptionally susceptible to disease because they are kept in overcrowded conditions and they are constantly highly stressed. Antibiotics help to keep sick animals alive long enough to be slaughtered and fed into the food chain. Antibiotics are also given because they help to stop diseases spreading quickly among animals who are kept in cramped and entirely unnatural conditions. When animals live in hideously confined quarters it is nigh on impossible to stop infections spreading without using antibiotics. Many American and European farmers routinely put antibiotics into the feed they give their animals to prevent infections developing. The antibiotics that are dished out in this grossly irresponsible way are often the same antibiotics that are becoming dramatically less effective in the treatment of human diseases.

But farmers don't just give antibiotics to animals in order to deal with disease. They also put antibiotics into their animal feed in order to promote growth. Antibiotics increase the muscle bulk of animals - and therefore increase their value and the farmer's eventual profit.

The process by which antibiotic resistance develops on farms is simple to explain. When animals are given antibiotics the bacteria in their intestines build up an immunity to those antibiotics. Those antibiotic-resistant organisms then pass on to farmers and others who have contact with the animals. They pass into the environment (even though most animals are denied access to fields, their faeces and urine still reach the environment when they are dumped onto fields or discharged into rivers). And, of course, the antibiotic-resistant organisms pass into the food chain directly when animals are killed, chopped up and eaten by humans. When milk in the USA was tested researchers identified 52 different antibiotic residues.

Between them, doctors and farmers have put us all at risk. Around the world, millions of innocent people will die because bugs have now acquired immunity to previously valuable antibiotics.

The problem is exacerbated because our hospitals are filthy and the people who staff them probably can't even spell hygiene. Having talked to many doctors and nurses I am convinced that most don't know the basic principles of how diseases are spread - and how they can be controlled. An unhealthy majority, for example, seemed unaware that there is an important difference between an `infectious' disease (spread through the environment - including by air) and a `contagious' disease (spread by contact). I quizzed a dozen doctors and nurses in one large NHS hospital, including several who had specific responsibilities for controlling the spread of infections such as MRSA and C.difficile and none of them seemed to understand the basic principles of disease spread. Quite senior NHS personnel have tried to convince me that gastrointestinal infections are transmitted through the air and that this, not poor hygiene practises, explains why such bugs tend to sweep through hospital patients. When I produced evidence showing that they were wrong (although it is possible for bugs to be transmitted via an aerosol route the vast majority of infections are spread by poor hygiene) two members of NHS staff then tried to argue, apparently quite seriously, that bugs behaved differently in hospitals to the way they behaved elsewhere. One doctor insisted that bugs which are spread only by touch outside hospitals can be airborne inside hospitals. It is, perhaps, hardly surprising that staff don't bother to wash their hands and don't understand the importance of obeying the simplest rules about hygiene. And it is hardly surprising that the number of people dying from infections is rising dramatically. If you don't know how a disease is contracted you aren't likely to have much success in preventing its spread. Many doctors and nurses don't even seem to realise that common causes of vomiting, such as the norovirus, are spread largely through inadequate cleaning of contaminated wards.

I have, since the 1970s, been warning about the return of serious infections. The rise and rise of problems such as C.difficile and MRSA was quite predictable. And other bugs will come back in a big way too. In my book *Paper Doctors* (1977) I pointed out that two things would result in a rise in infectious diseases: a lack of hygiene in hospitals and the abuse of antibiotics. I also predicted the rise in antibiotic-resistant infections.

In practice, avoiding infections such as MRSA and C.difficile is not difficult. The best way to avoid them is to clean hospital wards and to persuade doctors, nurses and other members of staff to wash their hands in between seeing patients. But NHS hospitals are institutionally dirty. Public lavatories in France are cleaner than British hospitals. The area between beds is swept but the area under the beds is left dirty. Equipment is often filthy. Communal baths, showers and toilets are disgusting. Staff don't understand anything about hygiene. And no one cares.

Nothing is done about these problems because the complaints system is designed to protect the system rather than the patient. Hospitals are not interested in learning from their errors. They are only interested in denying the truth and avoiding responsibility. Medical records are kept not only to provide information but also with one eye on future litigation. One of the problems is that hospital staff (like other public service employees) are almost impossible to sack. When one former NHS chief executive was forced to resign her Ł150,000 a year job over Britain's deadliest superbug outbreak she demanded a Ł150,000 pay off. The woman left her job after at least 90 patients died from C.difficile. And shortly after leaving her NHS job she set up a healthcare consultancy company (presumably, to tell the NHS how to improve hospitals). (She set up the company with her partner who had quit a senior NHS job after the trust where he worked accumulated debts of Ł30 million.) It seems that those who do leave the NHS are well compensated for their failure. And the concept of `shame' seems as alien to the modern bureaucrat as the concept of `duty' or `responsibility'.

When the Healthcare Commission performed unannounced tests at 51 NHS Health Trusts they found that nine out of ten of them had failed to meet hygiene standards put in place to reduce hospital infections. Two out of three hospitals did not complete a deep clean of their wards before a deadline set by the Government.

The result is that thousands of patients die every year in NHS hospitals because patients acquire lethal but avoidable infections. No one ever apologises. It is rare for anyone to be disciplined. Drivers go to prison if they are convicted of dangerous driving so why don't hospital staff go to prison for dangerous practices? If they did then I suspect that there would be far fewer unnecessary deaths in our hospitals. Twice as many Britons are killed by hospital infections as are killed on the roads. The total number of deaths from hospital superbugs such as MRSA and C.difficile is now well over 5,000 a year. The reason? Filthy wards, unhygienic practices, scandalously poor cleaning, grubby operating theatres and staff who never wash their hands. There are more such infections in British hospitals than anywhere else in the world. Why? British hospitals are dirtier than hospitals anywhere else in the world. Why? The staff in British hospitals are the most incompetent hospital staff in the world.

When my mother was in the Royal Devon and Exeter Hospital I stood in a hospital corridor and watched an auxiliary wheel a food trolley into a room where a patient was being barrier nursed. Half a dozen nurses were standing just feet away from the auxiliary. Eating chocolates and chatting, they watched the auxiliary but either did not see what she was doing or did not care. It was as though the she did not exist. The auxiliary wheeled in the trolley, handed out the food, came out and continued around the ward. No gloves, no mask, no gown. And no protection for the trolley or the food. I wasn't the slightest bit surprised to read that a couple died after contracting C.difficile in Royal Devon and Exeter hospital. I'm afraid that my only surprise is that so many patients are still alive when they leave. The rise in the incidence of superbugs is a phenomenon almost unknown outside the NHS and in my opinion it is a direct result of poor management and appallingly low standards of nursing. In the Middle Ages patients used to keep out of hospitals whenever they could - knowing that a hospital stay could well prove fatal. Things aren't much different today. In my view the Royal Devon and Exeter (like many other hospitals) should have a Government health warning hanging over the front door. And the staff should have health warnings stamped on their foreheads. I wouldn't license the place as an abattoir.

Since Ignaz Philipp Semmelweiss first demonstrated (in the mid-19th century) that deaths in the delivery room were caused by dirty hands every child has been taught the importance of basic personal hygiene. Sadly, the message does not seem to have got through to the medical and nursing professions. Countless studies have shown that hospital staff just don't bother to wash their hands. A study of doctors' habits showed that two out of three anaesthetists failed to wash their hands before treating a new patient (even though anaesthetists frequently perform venepuncture surgery) while one in three surgeons did not wash their arms properly before an operation. At least one-third of all hospital infections are caused by dirty hands.

The cost of all this in simple financial terms is colossal. Treating hospital contracted infections uses up around 15% of the hospital budget in the UK and adds around a week to each patient's hospital stay. The cost in human terms is incalculable: tens of thousands of patients die because of bugs they've caught from doctors, nurses, other staff or contaminated equipment. These aren't statistics: they are people. Real people. Every one of those unnecessary deaths is someone's wife, husband, mother, father, son, daughter, uncle, aunt, friend or neighbour. And remember, most of those patients die because doctors and nurses can't be bothered to wash their hands properly or because operating theatres aren't properly cleaned between operations.

The medical answer is - surprise, surprise - often to prescribe antibiotics and a third of hospital patients end up taking them. It now takes 50 times as much penicillin to treat an infection as was required 30 years ago.

There is no doubt that antibiotic-resistant bacteria are now commoner in the UK because of the sloppiness in NHS hospitals as well as the bad prescribing habits of doctors.

It is hardly surprising that people who stay at home to be treated - or who go home quickly after day-case or short-stay surgery - usually get better much quicker than people who need long-stay treatment and who have to go into hospital.

It is because NHS hospitals are so filthy that there are more food related infections in the NHS than in the seediest, most disreputable restaurants. Hospitals which are home to rats and cockroaches (as many NHS hospitals are) are an excellent breeding ground for bugs of all sorts. Dirty hospitals are dirty because they are badly managed and because the staff are lazy or incompetent.

Attempts to deal with this embedded problem range between pathetic and laughable. An NHS hospital in Buckinghamshire was reported to have recorded a rap song to help staff learn how to wash their hands. The song apparently included the lyrics: `Now clean between your fingers, just in case the bad bug lingers'. The hospital produced a video in which nurses wearing back to front baseball caps and bling jewellery stamped along to the beat. This was not a Xmas party joke and nor was it intended for children. This was a serious attempt to teach NHS staff how to wash their hands.

Nurses have even called for a vaccine to stop hospital infections spreading. It is, I suppose, easier to give a vaccine than to wash your hands.

The real problem is that hospital staff just don't seem to understand how infections spread. For example, it is common to see nurses in shops still wearing their uniforms, complete with dubious looking stains. Nurses who wear their uniforms out of the hospital environment are showing just how ignorant they are. Bugs are transferred both ways. Nurses bring dangerous antibiotic-resistant bacteria out into the community and they take infections back into the hospital with them. Nursing staff should change their clothes whenever they leave the hospital where they work. And doctors working in hospital should always wear freshly laundered white coats. (I did not wear a white coat when I worked as a GP because I always thought it acted as a barrier between myself and my patients. But GPs are not usually involved with patients leaking blood, pus and faeces.)

There is now no doubt that infections are a major killer in our State hospitals. Watch the cleaners at work and you'll see them slide a mop down the centre of the ward. It's known in the mop wielding business as `taking the mop for a walk'. They then wander off into their staff room for a tea break. And then serve patients their food. Staggeringly, the same people who clean the ward then serve patients their food. No one seems to see anything odd in this. The cleaners do not, of course, wash their hands between these two activities. Cleaning staff (sorry, I think they now have to be called `housekeepers') do not appear to have been told that they too must obey the basic rules of hygiene. The Government would save far more lives if it took down speed cameras and, instead, put up cameras in hospitals to check that nurses, cleaners and doctors wash their hands properly. Such a simple action would save billions of pounds and thousands of lives a year. Nurses who are spotted moving from patient to patient without washing their hands should be fired and banned from ever working in health care again.

The bad news is that things are going to get much, much worse I'm afraid. If Health and Safety operatives really want to save lives they should stop worrying about irrelevant `health threats' and concentrate all their efforts on NHS hospitals. Meanwhile, when patients die because of superbugs why aren't the doctors and nurses involved charged with manslaughter?

In the future two things are likely to happen.

First, the number of serious, deadly infections in our hospitals will rise. There will be periods when the infections will appear to be under control. But they will not be. Our hospital staff are institutionally lazy. Incompetence and ignorance are defended, protected and rewarded with promotion.

Second, the superbugs will escape from hospitals and start to kill people in their homes and places of work. It is already happening. Medical officers in Holland have found that 50% of Dutch farmers are carrying a new strain of MRSA that is passed from hormone-fed pigs to humans. Already, a new, more virulent strain of MRSA has been found in the community. And the number of elderly people killed in care homes by the superbug C.difficile has officially tripled in the last two years. (Since killer bugs are often not mentioned on death certificates the true figure is undoubtedly far higher than this.) This sad development is hardly surprising when one considers that nurses and local authority personnel who have responsibility for standards in care homes were trained in our hospitals.

In late 2008, a tiny report appeared in some newspapers headed 'Mutant superbug is found on farm'. Upon investigation it appeared that a superbug, a new variety of E.coli resistant to antibiotics had been found among cattle on a dairy farm in the north of England. It was, apparently the first time the particular strain of the bug had been found in Britain and it was only the third time the bug had ever been found anywhere in the world. A Government spokeswoman said that 'no additional precautions are warranted'.

23. The Cancer Industry: Misdirected And Ineffective

Cancer is, along with heart disease, stroke and doctors, one of the four big killers of our time. But cancer is the killer that frightens people most. The very word is so emotive that most doctors try not to use it when talking to patients. Instead of talking of cancer they talk of `tumours' and `growths'. They know that cancer is something most people don't even like to talk about.

Until it touches them or someone in their family most people try not to think about cancer. When they see a collecting tin for a cancer charity they may pop in a few coins in the belief that by making a donation to a cancer charity they are helping to conquer the disease. Putting money into a cancer charity collecting tin is like throwing coins into a wishing well; it is the 21st century equivalent of a good luck charm.

In order to ensure that money continues to pour in, the cancer industry must persuade potential contributors and supporters that it is making progress in the fight against cancer. Inevitably, the industry needs a vast quantity of money just to remain in business; there are salaries to be paid, rents and rates to be paid, electricity bills to be paid, advertising and public relations departments to pay for and so on.

To help in this aim the huge worldwide cancer industry must frequently release news about exciting new cancer remedies. Some of these widely promoted new treatments are in the early stages of being tested on human patients, some are not yet being tested on humans but are promoted as the new `wonder' cure for cancer on the basis of animal experiments, and some are talked about as new `breakthroughs' largely or even exclusively on the basis of a scientist's theory or hypothesis. These news stories raise hopes falsely and distract attention and finance from those areas which really need it (the prevention of cancer and the care of those who have cancer) but they serve the purpose: they raise money for the cash-hungry cancer industry.

When someone rattles a collecting tin in front of you and tells you that they need just a few more pence in order to continue with their breakthrough research it is difficult to say `no'. It is hardly surprising that the worldwide cancer industry's income continues to grow at a quite phenomenal rate.

But has the cancer industry really made any noticeable progress in the fight against cancer? I don't think so. The mortality figures show that more people are dying from commoner forms of cancer now than were a generation ago. One in three people already has, or will develop, cancer.

Today, despite the vast amounts of money spent on research, cancer is firmly positioned (along with circulatory disease and doctors) as one of the three big `killers' of the westernised world. The fact that the incidence of cancer has increased dramatically during the 20th and 21st centuries confirms, in my opinion, the view that cancer is, to a large extent, a man-made disease, created largely by our changing diet and our addiction to tobacco as well as our exposure to chemicals and pollution. Researchers found only one case of cancer among hundreds of Egyptian mummies and by the 19th century cancer was still a relatively uncommon disease. According to Garrison's *History of Medicine* the disease only began to show an `alarming increase' in the early part of the 20th century.

The incidence of cancer has steadily gone up despite or because of the absurdly named and poorly planned `war on cancer'. In my view the people who are well-paid to `fight' cancer have made things worse by desperately searching for cures instead of concentrating their efforts on dealing with identified causes. The trouble is that the cures they produce and promote (at such enormous profit) often make things worse, not better. In America it has been estimated that around $110 billion a year is spent on cancer. That is more than 10% of American's entire health care bill. But, in America, the incidence of cancer has steadily risen as has the number of people dying of cancer. The treatment methods of choice (surgery, chemotherapy and radiation therapy) have not improved mortality rates.

Scientists who have assessed the value of the war against cancer agree that we are losing the fight and that there is no evidence to suggest that decades of expensive research have had much, if any, effect on the most fundamental measure of success or failure - death. In areas where cancer has become more amenable to treatment, or now takes fewer lives, it is usually changes in lifestyle which are responsible - not discoveries made in the laboratory.

There are, I believe, several reasons why those fighting the war against cancer are losing. In my book *Paper Doctors* (published in 1977) I complained that: `Medical researchers involved in publicly or charitably financed cancer research persist in looking for the `magical cure'. Much laboratory work has been started on the mistaken assumption that there is one disease called `cancer' and that there will be a `cure' which will enable doctors to treat all the patients suffering with cancer. Many projects have been funded because organisers (both qualified and lay) believed that they might solve the problem of cancer once and for all to the well publicised credit of everyone concerned. Much money has undoubtedly been wasted on research which has duplicated work done elsewhere and which has moved in directions unlikely ever to prove of practical benefit.' The cancer industry still spends a vast fortune every year searching for the silver bullet.

Breast cancer is one of the most constantly publicised and most greatly feared forms of cancer. Because of its very nature it is a type of cancer which arouses much emotion. Newspapers, magazines and medical journals have for decades been full of articles describing new forms of treatment. The medical journal, *The Lancet*, in an editorial, commented that: `If one were to believe all the media hype, the triumphalism of the profession in published research, and the almost weekly miracle breakthroughs trumpeted by the cancer charities, one might be surprised that women are dying at all from this cancer.'

The lies, deceits and myths about the cancer industry are nowhere better illustrated than by breast cancer. In February 2011, it was reported that the incidence of breast cancer was rising. And at roughly the same time it was finally, officially, admitted that breast cancer is caused by diet. Anyone who has studied the causes of breast cancer would not find this difficult to understand.

For over two decades I have been pointing out that the evidence proves that breast cancer (probably above all others) is linked directly to diet and, in particular, to the consumption of cheap, fatty meat. My attempts to publicise this proven truth have been made infinitely more difficult by organisations such as the Advertising Standards Authority (which banned advertisements for my book *Food for Thought* because it truthfully linked cancer to meat consumption) and the Press Complaints Commission (which rolled over obediently when asked to do so by the meat trade and condemned me for publicising the truth about the meat-cancer link).

Since 1942 there has been steadily accumulating evidence to show that there is a link between breast cancer and dietary fat. I have little doubt that breast cancer could have been turned into a relatively uncommon disease, instead of one of the major killers of women, if politicians and doctors had been prepared to take on the food industry - and force the cancer industry to spread the truth. The American National Academy of Sciences, has concluded that `cancers of most major sites are influenced by dietary factors'. It has been estimated that `a little more than 40% of cancers in men and almost 60% of cancers in women in the United States could be attributed to dietary factors'.

Despite the quantity of epidemiological evidence which is available to show that fat and breast cancer are linked no one really knows the mechanism through which fat causes cancer. One theory is that synthetic chemicals - commonly used in the manufacture of pesticides - concentrate in the fatty tissues of animals. People who then eat bits and pieces of dead animal absorb the synthetic chemicals into their own bodies - and the concentrations of chemicals steadily rise. (In an average lifetime a meat eater will consume 36 pigs, 36 sheep, 750 chickens and turkeys and several cows.) More than 177 organochlorines (synthetic chemicals created when chlorine gas is bonded to carbon-rich organic matter) have been found in the tissues of the general population of the United States and Canada. Organochlorines can cause infertility, birth defects, miscarriages, immune system suppression, metabolic dysfunction, behavioural disorders, hormonal abnormalities and cancer.

These chlorine based compounds can cause cancer in various ways. Some cause cancer directly. Others produce cancers by interfering with or mimicking human hormones. A third group suppress the immune system and then enhance the carcinogenic effect of other chemicals. These chemicals seem to strike first at the reproductive system - which is probably why a heavy fat consumption increases the risk of developing cancers of the breast, prostate, and uterus.

We accept chemicals because they make our life easier, and because the big chemical companies have become financially and politically powerful. We assume that they are essential and we assume that they are safe because that is what the big companies tell us. I don't believe they are essential and I certainly don't believe that they are safe. There is no little irony in the fact that the pharmaceutical industry makes billions of dollars selling drugs for the treatment of cancers which some believe may have been created by its billion dollar sister industry: the chemical industry.

Convincing epidemiological evidence has been collected by the journal *Australasian Health and Healing* to support the theory that it is the chemicals in fat which cause cancer. Women in parts of America which were routinely blanketed with aerial sprayings of the pesticide DDT during the 1950s have one of the highest rates of breast cancer in America. Female chemical workers who were exposed to high levels of dioxin in a German pesticide plant had double the cancer mortality rate of the German population - and higher than average rates of breast cancer. A study in America produced similar results. Women professional golfers, most of whom play the game every day, have a high rate of breast cancer. It is suspected that these women may have been poisoned by the chemicals with which most golf courses are saturated. According to a U.S. Environmental Protection Agency study, parts of America with hazardous waste sites are 6.5 times as likely to have a high breast cancer rate than other areas. Women who have breast cancer have high blood levels of the chemicals suspected of causing the disease. A study of 229 women from New York City showed that women who developed breast cancer had substantially higher levels of suspected pesticide chemicals. During the early 1970s breast cancer rates in Israel were among the highest and fastest rising in the world. In 1978, Israel phased out the use of several suspected pesticides. Doctors noted that the levels of chemicals in breast milk dropped quite quickly. The incidence of breast cancer duly started to fall too.

But how many doctors now advocate a low fat, meat free diet for women who are regarded as susceptible to breast cancer? Very few. Most prefer to prescribe drugs or to recommend the surgical removal of healthy breasts. Where, sadly, is the financial profit opportunity in merely recommending a dietary change?

There has been much talk of a breast cancer gene (BRCA-1) but there isn't really any such thing. There is no gene which *causes* breast cancer. There is, however, a gene which increases a woman's chances of developing cancer. Women with this gene can dramatically reduce their risk of developing breast cancer by avoiding the factors which are known to be associated with breast cancer. They should, for example, avoid becoming overweight, cut out meat completely and eat a low fat diet. Women who are overweight have more fat in their bodies and are more likely to develop cancer of the breast. The modern `scientific' approach (to remove the healthy breasts of women who have the breast cancer gene) is barbaric and unnecessary.

Perhaps the biggest irony of all is the fact that although doctors have widely ignored the available evidence that would have enabled them to protect most of their patients from breast cancer (and, indeed, many other major types of cancer too) they have devised their own high technology form of preventive medicine - the mammogram. It is difficult not to be cynical about this. Teaching women how to reduce their chances of developing breast cancer (and teaching them how to check their own breasts for lumps) would earn the profession very little. So the medical profession and its companion industries have introduced a high technology form of cancer detection so that they can make money out of the general anxiety about breast cancer. (I deal with mammograms in the section of this book dealing with `screening programmes'.)

In my book *2020* (published in 2010) I forecast that the incidence of breast cancer in China would rise. It was not a difficult prediction. The Chinese people, growing in wealth, are dramatically increasing their intake of meat. When the same thing happened in Japan a few years ago the result was a dramatic increase in the incidence of breast cancer in Japanese women. The ones who stuck to a low-meat traditional Japanese diet were far less likely to develop breast cancer when compared to the women who changed to a high-meat American style diet. Just a little more than a year after I wrote *2020* it was revealed that my prediction was already coming true.

The meat sold today causes far more cancer than ever before because it is very fatty and full of carcinogens. There are two reasons for this. First, farmers who sell heavy, fatty animals get more money for them. Second, farmers use carcinogenic chemicals on their farms. And those chemicals end up in the animal's fat.

It is these two facts which explain why the incidence of cancer always rises when populations start eating more meat.

But why is the incidence of breast cancer particularly likely to rise?

The answer to that is simple too.

When animals eat toxic substances such as chemicals which are carcinogenic which have been sprayed on the grass or put into the food they eat, the chemicals are stored in their fatty tissues. The fattier the animal is the more carcinogens it will have stored in its body. And, when it is killed and eaten, those carcinogens will be consumed by the person eating the meat. And, as with animals, the carcinogens will tend to gravitate to, and be stored in, the fatty tissues.

Breasts contain a good deal of fat. There is remarkably little actual breast tissue in a breast. Most of the breast is fat. And the bigger the breast the more fat there is likely to be. This is why breast cancer is commoner among older women. They tend to have more fat on their bodies in general and to have bigger and fattier breasts in particular. Poorer people tend to eat fattier meat. That's why poor people tend to get more cancer than rich people.

I first put forward this theory in an early (and now out of print) book of mine called *Power Over Cancer*. No one has ever disputed my conclusions. However, instead of discouraging women from eating meat, doctors prefer to remove healthy breasts from women considered genetically susceptible to breast cancer in order to prevent them getting breast cancer.

We don't need more money pouring into cancer research because we already know what causes most forms of cancer. According to one honest observer: `Basic cancer research is an excellent slush fund for molecular biologists but it won't have any impact on cancer'. Cancer is created by chemical pollutants, by unhealthy, fatty, food and by tobacco. Poisoned water supplies, dangerous prescription drugs and the overuse of X-rays have also contributed to the incidence of cancer.

With immune systems constantly battered by polluted air, adulterated and chemically impregnated food and a constant onslaught from the drugs we buy for ourselves, or allow our doctors to prescribe for us, it is not surprising that increasing numbers of people succumb to one of the many different types of cancer. We know what causes 80% of all cases of cancer. Eight out of ten people who develop cancer could have been saved if money and effort had been put into prevention.

I do not believe that any wonder cure for cancer will come from the `cancer industry'. But if I had the annual income the cancer industry enjoys I believe that I could turn cancer into a historical oddity within five years.

'Why,' you may ask, 'do the big cancer charities not spend more money on trying to prevent cancer? Why do they spend all their money gambling on the chance of finding a `cure' when they could save millions of lives simply by using their resources to publicise what we already know?'

To understand the answers to these questions you have to understand that, as I have indicated, the cancer research industry is exactly that - an industry. It is a massive, worldwide multi-billion dollar industry which employs hundreds of thousands of scientists and administrators. Sadly, I suspect that for many of these employees the search for a cure for cancer has become the end instead of just the beginning. Much of the cancer industry is run by and for scientific researchers. The cancer industry needs a constant stream of dollars to keep its laboratories running. If the cancer industry spent its income on explaining to people how to avoid cancer there would be little or no place for research laboratories and a great many scientists would be put out of work. Worse still, if the cancer industry reduced the number of people dying of cancer its own income would fall.

Besides, those whose job it is to raise money know that it is far easier to persuade people to put money into a collecting tin if you tell them that they are contributing towards the search for a cure. Persuading people to avoid known causes of cancer is thankless work. Not many people will put money into your collecting tin if you stand on a street corner handing out leaflets containing sensible eating advice. It is much easier to raise money if you talk about new breakthroughs and show photographs of people (preferably children or pretty young women) who are dying of cancer. It is much easier to raise a million dollars for a new piece of machinery than it is to raise a million dollars for a print bill or a television advertising campaign designed to explain to people how they can avoid cancer.

Those who are responsible for raising money for the cancer industry know that it is impossible to personalise a preventive medicine campaign because you can never show a picture of a man, woman or child whose life has been saved by a leaflet. A picture of a child who is dying of cancer and who is waiting for laboratory scientists to find a cure will attract far more public support than an appeal for funds to help save unnamed individuals in the future.

And so it is the scientists searching for laboratory cures who get the big grants and the prestigious awards and who are fussed over and praised by the politicians and the journalists. Scientists who have established links which would enable us to save millions of lives by organising effective prevention programmes are as unlikely to win Nobel prizes as are doctors who devote themselves to teaching the principles of healthy living to millions of people.

There are many explanations for this disastrous misreading of the needs within cancer research. Undoubtedly one important reason is that there are thousands of surgeons, radiologists and radiotherapists (not to mention pure researchers) earning their living from traditional methods of cancer research and control. Public health is not a fashionable speciality within the medical profession: there is no opportunity for private practice and a general lack of financial incentive for brighter physicians to enter this field. And of equal importance perhaps is the fact that industrial pressures all oppose attempts to control the causative factors responsible for the vast majority of cancers.

Today, the cancer researchers are still pleading for more money (as they have been doing for decades); they are still promising that if they are given enough money they will be able to find a cure for cancer. It is, they suggest, only a shortage of money which is responsible for the continuing rise in the incidence of cancer deaths. They want to do more animal experiments and they have now devised animals which are genetically bred to develop cancer.

Cancer industry employees say they want to know `how' cancer develops. They don't seem to understand that the `how' is not important. It would be nice to know the `how'. But it is the `why' which matters. And we already know why cancer is a major killer. By insisting on finding the `how' the cancer industry is playing right into the hands of the industries which are responsible for much cancer. The tobacco industry is constantly calling for more research into the links between tobacco and cancer. By calling for more research the tobacco industry is able to make itself look good - and at the same time to suggest that there is still some controversy and doubt about the links between tobacco and cancer.

But we don't need more research into tobacco and cancer. Everything we need to know can be summed up in four words: `Smoking tobacco causes cancer.' And all we need now is a proper programme to persuade people not to smoke. But Governments continue to spend millions fighting an unwinnable `drugs war' against the users of cannabis, cocaine and heroin while they subsidise tobacco - a much more dangerous drug.

The tobacco industry isn't the only industry trying to cause confusion and doubt. Every cancer producing industry follows the same route: campaigning for more and more research and claiming that it is research and not prevention which will lead to a solution.

Consumers quite like the idea of someone finding a `cure' for cancer because it means that they can carry on eating the fatty food they like and smoking the cigarettes they enjoy without having to worry. `Had such campaigns been at work during the Irish potato famine, which killed more than a million Irish between 1845 and 1849, they might have engendered studies into the biomechanical processes of famine rather than the social forces that gave rise to it,' wrote Robert N. Proctor in *The Sciences*. `Investigators would have secured funding for research into why starvation ran in families instead of examining the social Darwinist policies of the Manchester era or studying how Ireland was able to export grain even during the worst years of the famine.'

There are very few industries in the world which have grown as rapidly as the cancer industry - the charities, laboratories, research scientists and administrators who are devoted to the search for a cure for cancer have, in recent years, spent billions.

But the irony is the fact that money really isn't the key issue. You cannot `buy' successful research. Although the huge cancer industry has spent a vast portion of its massive budget on laboratory research designed to find a `magic' cure for cancer the majority of the most important and dramatic discoveries about cancer have been made by observant practitioners who have devoted themselves to a study of human patients and their habits.

In my book *Paper Doctors* (1977) I explained: `One of the most important breakthroughs in cancer research of recent years was made, not by researchers in expensive institutes but by a practising British surgeon, Denis Burkitt, working in Uganda. His first research grant from Government funds totalled Ł15 and his second, for Ł150, came from the Medical Research Council and was spent on an old jeep. By logical, patient study Burkitt managed to map the occurrence of a tumour common in children in that part of the world. He matched the map he prepared with other factors and eventually managed to show that the cancer was probably caused by a virus. Eventually he learnt how to cure the tumour. So, one of the most important discoveries was made, not by a professional researcher but by an observant doctor happy to continue his studies in his own time and at his own expense. Too many doctors these days are unwilling to begin any research programme unless they are first financed by an official agency and properly recognised as bona fide research workers.'

There have been some very important advances in cancer treatment in recent years. But they have been largely limited to rare cancers that tend to occur in children and young adults, and those make up only perhaps one or two per cent of the total cancer burden. Cancer death rates continue to go up year after year. And survival rates are no better today than they were. The cancer industry deliberately draws attention to its modest successes in the treatment of a few, relatively uncommon childhood cancers (putting pictures of children whose lives have been saved onto promotional leaflets and posters is a sure-fire way to keep the money pouring in). But there has been little or no improvement in the death rates for the big killers: lung cancer, breast cancer, prostate cancer or cancer of the colon.

None of this explains why Governments have also failed to teach their citizens the facts about cancer. However, there are, I believe, two explanations for this seemingly mysterious state of affairs. Firstly, Governments are always wary of annoying big, powerful, tax-paying industries and there is absolutely no doubt that many huge, international corporations would be (to put it mildly) exceedingly upset if millions of potential consumers were warned of the dangers of eating meat. Secondly, (and I offer no excuse for the fact that this sounds extremely cynical) Governments do not want people to live longer. On the contrary, they have a vested interest in people not living too long. People who live on into their 60s, 70s and 80s have to be given pensions and cost Governments a great deal of money.

And, of course, doctors are educated by the drug industry, and controlled by it, and the result is that when the average doctor thinks of `patients' he or she thinks of `drugs'. Doctors are taught to respond to illness by prescribing a bottle or a packet of pills. Most doctors have been so brainwashed by the powerful international drugs industry that they regard any treatment which does not involve drugs as hocus pocus and they regard preventive medicine as trivial, irrelevant nonsense which is rather beneath them. And so, for doctors, cancer means chemotherapy.

Doctors frequently claim that people who reject chemotherapy do so because they are fearful of the side effects. This is simplistic and inaccurate and bears comparison with the erroneous claim that people emigrate simply because they want better weather. Patients reject chemotherapy for many reasons. Some know that chemotherapy may damage their recovery and speed their demise. And some know that chemotherapy is grossly overrated, simply does not work and is, like radiotherapy, often likely to do more harm than good. But the slightly sneery accusation that patients who reject chemotherapy do so because they are frightened of the side effects is demeaning, patronising and unworthy. It is also typical of the apologists who defend the drug industry at any cost and who always put the defence of the industry above their compassion and understanding for patients.

The British Government has introduced a Ł2 billion cancer scheme to help patients but most of the money has been wasted on yet more bureaucracy. Around 400 new administrative posts have been created, with administrative officers paid around Ł40,000 a year each. The result of all this misdirection of resources is that Britain still has one of the worst cancer survival rates in Western Europe. In the UK, 36% of men with cancer are likely to live beyond 5 years. This compares very badly with figures of 45% in France and Germany, 50% in Sweden and 55% in Austria.

Finally, it is worth remembering that we know what causes 80% of all cancers. If people ate less fatty food and avoided meat, the incidence of cancer would plummet.

24. Travelling For Treatment

For as long as it continues to exist, the NHS will continue to decline. Moreover, private care (currently providing the sort of level of service provided by the NHS two or three decades ago) will also deteriorate. Many consultants who were previously working exclusively in the NHS have carried their bad manners into private practice and many patients don't know enough to expect better. Even private hospitals have deteriorated, because of the appalling standard set by the NHS. Visit a private hospital and the chances are that you will sit in a crowded waiting room. After a lengthy wait you will be hurried in to see your consultant who will rush through your consultation so that she (or he) can get onto the next patient. `Payment in advance please, please see the receptionist. Cash, cheques and all major credit cards taken.' Private patients now routinely have to wait days (or weeks) to receive the results of simple blood tests, X-ray tests or tissue sample tests. And they have to wait weeks (or months) for essential, life-saving surgery. Paying privately in Britain now buys you better food, slightly more polite nurses and a television set all of your own that you don't have to feed with tokens. But it doesn't buy you better medical care (which is, I suspect, what most people suspect they're going to get when they spend vast amounts of money on private health insurance) though it does, importantly, buy you a good chance of avoiding a deadly antibiotic-resistant infection.

Normal health care practice in other countries is to receive test results within an hour or so and, if you have a serious disorder needing treatment, to receive that within a few days. Not even private patients get that level of care in Britain today. So, not surprisingly, a growing number of Britons now go abroad for health care; travelling to India or Thailand for medical and surgical treatment. Hospitals in these countries are far cleaner, far more modern and far better equipped than British hospitals. Patients go to hospitals and clinics in Poland, Bulgaria and Japan. And they go not just because they can avoid long waiting lists or because private hospital care is much cheaper than it is in the UK but because they know that they will be treated better and they will be safer. There is far less risk of infection in most other countries. Patients go abroad for major operations and they go for the treatment of relatively minor ailments; many even go abroad for dental treatment.

And the prices (which often include first class hotel accommodation for accompanying relatives) are, even when the costs of travel are included, often considerably lower than the price of treatment in the UK. For example, in the early summer of 2011 the price of a cataract removal in the UK was listed at Ł2,175. The same operation would cost Ł490 in Bulgaria. A coronary bypass would cost Ł13,650 in the UK and Ł4,721 in India. A hip replacement would cost Ł9,500 in the UK and Ł2,900 in Tunisia. A full set of dentures which would cost Ł565 in the UK would cost Ł156 in Latvia. The private surgery prices in the UK are high because NHS waiting lists are deliberately manipulated, and cruelly long, and private hospitals and doctors take advantage of the demand by pushing their prices sky high. (In the summer of 2011, it was announced that some Primary Care Trusts within the NHS were imposing minimum waiting times in the hope that at least some of the patients waiting for treatment would either die or choose to pay for private treatment.)

Patients travel abroad not just because operations and treatments are cheaper outside the UK (and do not involve a long waiting time) but also because they know that the medical and nursing care will be far superior, that they will receive better food and that their relatives will be better received. How embarrassing it is to have to write that. Some hospitals in the Far East have turned non-emergency, elective surgery into a quasi-holiday experience.

The quality of medical care in Britain will continue to deteriorate because the answer to all the bad things that happen is not to train people better (or, heaven forbid, to punish the worst offenders) but to add another layer of impenetrable bureaucracy, separating the people with the power from the people making the decisions, and to ensure that no one can ever be held responsible for anything they do. The people with the power protect the lowly people who take the decisions because that helps to protect the position of the people with the power. It's an unwritten rule. No one must be punished or even reprimanded because once you start down that slippery slope you end up with some higher level official having to accept responsibility and that cannot be contemplated. And so nothing ever improves. Problems merely create more cover ups. The only concern is to avoid anyone having to say `sorry', or admit that they have made a mistake. Patients and their relatives may remain unsatisfied, aggrieved or concerned that someone else will suffer in exactly the same way that they did. But none of this seems to matter as long as no jobs are lost or even threatened. Hospital bureaucrats prefer to pay off a litigant (without admitting liability or having to resign) than to defend a case in court.

25. Cockroaches With Computers

In the bad old days when I was a young doctor, and doctors and nurses were in charge of health care, hospitals were run by a matron. The administration would be managed by a hospital secretary (usually a weedy, almost invisible accountant assisted by a couple of typists and a filing clerk) and there would be a clerk on every ward who was responsible for filing the mail, the laboratory reports and the medical notes. The ward clerk would keep all the patients' records up-to-date and neatly filed in a little cabinet. (These days, wards have a row of administrators. Four or five of them sit there constantly scribbling. There are no nurses. Just clerks sitting scribbling. What are they all writing? I have no idea. But I can tell you that whatever it is it is bound to be unnecessary, self-serving guff.)

Today, hospitals are overrun with administrators. There are now more administrators in British hospitals than there are nurses. There are more administrators than beds, for heaven's sake. Commercial organisations everywhere are getting rid of middle managers by the lorry load and replacing them with computers; the NHS stands alone in acquiring more administrators as well as tons of computers. When my mother was being thrown out of hospital because she was only terminally ill and not finally terminally ill I attended two meetings. One meeting was attended by nine NHS employees who were there to insist that my mother be ejected from the hospital. The other meeting was held in an entirely empty hospital ward. `We don't have any beds,' said one of the NHS employees. `We have to discharge your mother.' It didn't seem to occur to her that they had plenty of beds - there were a stack of them in the room where we were having the meeting. And if they fired some of the bureaucrats they would have had plenty of money to hire any extra nurses they needed. Endless hours are wasted on meetings where people who have never met the patient and who know nothing about making a diagnosis, or arranging treatment, give their views about what should and should not be done. Organising meetings is the one thing the NHS does well. Large, bureaucratic organisations exist for meetings and Britain's National Health Service is the world's third largest employer (after the Chinese army and the Indian railways). The meetings, organised by bureaucrats, nurses and social workers are an end not a beginning. They provide a sense of importance and a reason for their own existence. The short-term aim is not to make decisions but, rather, to avoid making any decisions. The long-term aim is to ensure that another meeting can be arranged, the sense of self-importance sustained and the responsibility for making the wrong decision avoided.

Our hospitals are overrun with administrators and they are appalling. Are the two facts linked? You bet they are. Governments have repeatedly promised to get rid of mixed-sex wards. They've failed to manage even that. Today, Britain is one of the few countries in the world where men and women must share a ward and a bathroom. Even Third World countries have banished mixed-sex wards but NHS administrators, far too busy choosing biscuits for their next meeting, found it just too difficult. Doctors and nurses (who could have used their professional power to put an end to this but who have preferred to use their power only to improve their own financial circumstances) should cringe in shame and embarrassment. But I don't expect many will.

NHS hospitals are filthy. The food is inedible. Patients are treated with neither respect nor dignity. Doctors are hardly ever seen. Nurses are lazy. A Tory peer who was treated in an NHS hospital described his nurses as `grubby, drunken, promiscuous and lazy'. Charles Dickens' wonderful creation, Mrs Gamp, would have fitted into the modern NHS very well. NHS hospitals are as dangerous today as they were in the Middle Ages. The chances of a patient leaving an NHS hospital in better health than they were when they entered it are not high. The inescapable conclusion is that hospitals are run for the benefit not of patients but of the staff.

Everything in the NHS moves frighteningly slowly, and with scant regard for the welfare of patients. When it was announced in January 2009 that the World Health Organisation had devised a simple checklist which had been proved to cut surgical deaths by more than 40% and surgical complications by over a third, hospitals in England and Wales were ordered to use the checklist by February 2010. In other words, the Government allowed hospitals 13 months to adopt a simple checklist system. Is this what we have become? Is this the world we have created for ourselves? A bureaucracy so powerful that it takes 13 months to photocopy a list?

The money poured into the NHS in recent years could have been spent on providing the population with an endless supply of cocktail umbrellas for all the good it has done. A recent survey of more than 3,000 doctors showed that the majority believe that the Labour Government utterly failed to improve hospitals despite doubling the amount of taxpayers' money spent on them.

The problem, of course, is the bureaucracy. The figures aren't a secret. The main job of all the damned bureaucrats is to defraud the public and to ensure that the NHS doesn't waste good money on looking after patients. Money not wasted on patients can be spent on office equipment, weekend junkets and better expense accounts. If a revived Gestapo ever starts recruiting in the UK they would have little trouble in finding suitable candidates among the administrators working for the NHS.

And so thanks to the cruelty of the bureaucrats, and the self-centred blindness of doctors and nurses, the result is a patchy, unfair, destructive, lethal system which kills more people than it saves.

My wife needed a test which for unexplained political reasons could not be done at the hospital to which she had been referred. So the hospital she had visited sent four copies of the same letter through the post. One copy went to the doctor working at the first hospital, one copy went to the doctor at the second hospital, one copy went to my wife's doctor and one copy went to my wife. The second hospital then sent a copy of the same letter through the post to my wife's GP asking for an official referral letter. Copies of this letter went by post to the consultant at the first hospital (who had never actually seen my wife), the hospital records department at the first hospital, another department in the second hospital and my wife. Weeks later we all had lots of paperwork but there was still no sign of an appointment.

Because of the hordes of unnecessary bureaucrats, the NHS is now dangerously overstaffed. Billions of pounds are wasted on salaries, expenses and pensions for unnecessary administrators; an overpaid, cumbersome burden weighs down every part of the health service, discouraging and disrupting the work of doctors and nurses. Those excess administrators are soaking up so much money that they are indirectly responsible for thousands of deaths. A spokesman for one hospital which had spent Ł1,000,000 more than its budget allowed said that the hospital was `thinking' about what to do (putting it this way enables the administrators to avoid responsibility) and that what had happened was no one's fault (see what I mean). She said that the hospital was considering selling some equipment or closing some beds in order to deal with its debts. The hospital was not, of course, contemplating getting rid of any of the administrators whose incompetence had led to the problem. Most administrators seem to believe that hospitals would be much more efficient and cost effective if there were no patients at all. Signs of administrators at work are everywhere. For example, it is the fashion these days to put carpets on hospital corridors. Naturally, this is dangerously unhealthy (since carpets are far more difficult to clean than other forms of flooring) but at least it means that administrators are not disturbed by the noise of patients being wheeled about.

Today, Britain's National Health Service employs 1.4 million people. During the last decade or so the workforce has increased by nearly a quarter of a million. But there are less people actually caring for patients than there were a decade or so ago.

In an ideal world hospitals would be run by doctors - the only people working in hospital who have taken an Oath to care for their patients. But hospitals are now run by administrators and so doctors must do what they are told. The NHS has become a bonanza for bureaucrats. More than 60% of NHS employees are pen pushers. The NHS has been damaged beyond repair by a combination of factors but one primary problem has, for years, been the fact that NHS hospitals have always been absurdly over-endowed with two unnecessary life forms: cockroaches and administrators. It can, I suppose, be argued that the cockroaches are useful because they eat up bits of food that have been dropped on the floor. The administrators, however, are destructive, deadly and entirely without value. They contribute nothing to the welfare of patients but cost billions.

We should fire at least half of all NHS administrators immediately (it doesn't matter which half) and then sack half of the remainder (again, it doesn't matter which half). We should then give the remaining bureaucrats responsibility to match their authority. We should put an administrator on every ward - with responsibility for maintaining patients' records. This would free nurses to look after patients. Outside hospitals all patients should keep their own medical records. This would enable them to take their records to whichever doctor they were seeing - whether in general practice or in hospital.

The separation of authority from responsibility, and the devolution of clinical power, means that doctors are no longer in charge of what happens to their patients. Doctors work in teams (as equal members alongside such dross as social workers) led by administrators. Today, it is the administrators who are in charge. And administrators are, it seems, unsackable. Whenever a hospital runs short of money it is the facilities for patients which are cut - never the number of overpaid, underworked administrators. It is difficult to avoid the conclusion that modern hospitals and health centres are run for employees in general, and administrators in particular, rather than for patients. There are no penalties for bureaucrats who make a real mess of things. In December 2008 it was announced that Ł327,000,000 of debt would be wiped from ten hospital trusts that were in severe financial trouble. There was not, of course, any suggestion that any of the bureaucrats responsible would lose their jobs. In an average sort of year the NHS loses Ł500,000,000 a year as foreign Governments fail to reimburse it for treating foreigners who fell ill while holidaying in Britain. At the same time Britain pays out vast sums to cover the costs of British tourists treated in Europe. Is it beyond the wit of NHS bureaucrats to work out a way to hold back some of the money we pay out and put it against the money we are owed?

It is vital to get rid of bureaucrats not just because of the cost but because, in order to justify their existence, they need constantly to interfere. They deliberately complicate systems which work well and they work unceasingly to justify their importance, their huge salaries, their deputies, their assistants, their teams of secretaries and their spacious offices. Bureaucrats exist to acquire power and to avoid making decisions (which, in any case, they are not qualified to make). Administrators ensure that doctors are sucked into their system of time-wasting committees and meetings. Their whole purpose is control and the purpose of that is power and the purpose of that is money. The vast majority of NHS administrators are poor quality, badly trained, inadequately supervised and wildly overpaid. Bureaucrats are not just expensive; they are also destructive. In an ideal world over 90% of hospital administrators would spend their days wandering the streets dressed only in those indecent, humiliating, degrading, tie-at-the-back-and-show-the-world-your-bum gowns that hospitals force patients to wear.

When NHS bureaucrats decide what is good for people they take no notice of what people want or need. Bureaucrats live on meetings, like vampires live on blood, and so although they never want to make major changes they are always endeavouring to change the existing ways of doing things; causing curiously significant disruptions which benefit only themselves.

A friend of ours needed a new hearing aid because her old one had stopped working. But she couldn't have a new one unless her GP referred her afresh to the hospital. So she had to start again. Her GP had to refer her a second time. There was, inevitably, lots more paperwork and lots more administration. That's what the NHS is all about: paperwork and administration.

The world is full of rules and regulations and the world of medicine is no exception. But, in the medical world, they are always the wrong rules and regulations because they are created not to protect people but to protect the establishment; to protect bureaucrats, politicians, drug companies and the health professions.

26. Profits In Poor Countries

Although it is firmly based in the developed part of the world, the international drug industry happily makes whatever profits it can in the developing countries, marketing its products as unscrupulously as the tobacco giants.

Drug companies prefer to make (and sell) drugs which are prescribed for chronic illnesses common in rich countries. These drugs will need to be taken for years. It is for this reason that there are many drugs for psychiatric problems, high blood pressure, heart disease, arthritis, thrombosis, osteoporosis, pain relief, high cholesterol, obesity, sex problems and baldness. Vaccines are best of all because they can be given to millions of people around the world - even healthy people can be given vaccines. The drug companies sell 80% of their drugs in America, Europe and Japan. And they go to extraordinary lengths to please their customers (and enhance their profits). Drug companies can now put electronic markers into drug capsules. The marker sends a message to a sensor to remind patients if they miss a dose of their drug. How absurd and expensive. Why should doctors pander to laziness and stupidity in such a way?

Most drug companies look for products with a minimum sales potential of $500 million a year. This means that they make many drugs for the treatment of diseases which affect patients in rich countries and very few drugs for diseases which affect patients in poor countries.

Although drug companies spend virtually no money on studying the sort of diseases which afflict human beings in the developing countries they do, nevertheless, sell around 20% of the value of their drugs to the Governments of those countries. The drug companies will admit that diseases which afflict the people of Africa and Asia aren't profitable enough to merit any research investment but they will happily sell their expensive brand name versions of tranquillisers, sleeping tablets, painkillers, and the other pharmacological garbage of the developed world into those countries. Moreover, when they sell into developing countries the drug companies, like the tobacco companies, often use advertising and marketing techniques which not even the lax Governments of the West would allow. Indeed, they don't just sell products which are too dangerous for sale in the developed countries but they also use drugs in ways that would never be allowed in developed countries. For example, doctors in developing countries may be encouraged to prescribe drugs to help improve the growth of malnourished children who really just need enough food.

There is a ruthlessness about the drug companies which makes the arms business look positively philanthropic. Drug companies have even been known to push up prices of drugs in small developing countries which have been hit by epidemics. To the drug industry profit is everything.

27. Who Lives, Who Dies?

It is probably not widely known, but NHS staff frequently make decisions about which patients will be saved and which will be allowed to die. There aren't enough resources to provide for everyone in need. The rules which have to be followed mean that people with children take precedence over people who don't have children. So a scrounger who has never done a day's work in his life, but who has 12 kids, will take precedence over someone who works hard, pays taxes and plays an important role in society. The sensible and hard-working always lose out in every conceivable way. I have a vision that before long the NHS will introduce a reality television programme called *Who lives? Who dies? You decide?*. Twelve patients needing kidney transplants will all take part in the programme and `sell' themselves to the audience. The winner will receive the transplant and the NHS will keep all the phone line money. The awful, awful thing is that I cannot convince myself it could not happen.

28. Planning For Failure

Successive political administrations have recognised the need to streamline the NHS and have made the fundamental mistake of trying to improve things by fiddling with the structure. Naturally, the fiddling has, of course, always been done by administrators and has always resulted in the introduction of additional layers of administration.

No British Government seems constitutionally able to come into power without reorganising the NHS and so the organisation has steadily become increasingly bureaucratic with each change in administration; the layers just keep adding and the complexity grows. I have lost count of the number of times the NHS has been reorganised in my lifetime. The one thing I can guarantee is that every time they've reorganised it the administration has grown denser and more controlling. Albert Einstein knew what he was talking about when he said that: `Bureaucracy is the death of any achievement.' The tragedy is that in future there will be ever more reorganisation because the European Union has views on the provision of health care (as it does with everything else).

Naturally, the politicians always claim that they are making changes in order to improve things for patients but in practice they always do exactly the opposite because the administrators (who run the NHS and who decide what changes will be made) ensure that the end result of any reorganisation is not that things are made simpler but that yet another layer of administration is added. The one certainty in a bureaucratic organisation is that no administrator ever gets fired as a result of a reorganisation. It is an inevitable fact of life that every reorganisation of any large organisation run by the State will be bigger, more bureaucratic and less efficient at the end of the reorganisation than it was at the beginning. And the politicians (who have no idea how the NHS is organised) never dare to tackle the basic problem which is that the NHS itself is based upon an entirely false premise. And so, every reorganisation makes the bureaucracy bigger, more intrusive and more powerful and reduces the authority of doctors and the quality of the service patients receive.

The result is that today, the NHS, intrinsically corrupt and inefficient, would fit well into the old Soviet Union. I have been studying the NHS for over 40 years and know now that the big questions will never be addressed because it will always be inconvenient to do so. In any large organisation (and in Europe they don't come any larger than the NHS) employees are judged not by success but by the absence of failure. And in today's NHS things are worse than that in that failure is only failure if it is admitted and within the NHS failure is never admitted.

Every time there is a reorganisation patients are promised more freedom but every reorganisation means that patients have less freedom than they had before. They do not, for example, have real freedom of choice of doctor or hospital or remedy. This sort of basic freedom is essential but patients cannot see the doctor of their choice (as most would if they were paying direct). Instead, they see the doctor who is available (if there is a doctor available). In general practice, patients see the doctor to whom they have been allocated - or, rather, they are put under the care of a practice to which they have been allocated.

The people who make decisions about NHS cuts are the administrators - the people whose jobs ought to go but never do. Whenever cuts are made it is, of course, always nurses and doctors who go. The doctors and nurses who remain are forced by each new reorganisation to spend increasing amounts of their time on administration, attending wall to wall meetings and dealing with the odd patient here and there when time allows.

Politicians never have the sense, or the courage, to admit that the whole damned idea of the NHS was a bad one, and will never work satisfactorily from the patients' point of view. No one is ever prepared to admit that because a State-run system allies the medical profession and the State it isolates the patient. Politicians, drug companies, bureaucrats and staff all have a vested interest in maintaining the NHS beast. And the administrators are clever enough to ensure that the people who might make a fuss (the doctors) always come well out of any reorganisation. So, thanks to recent NHS reorganisations, GPs are today underworked and overpaid. They are paid better, for less work, than doctors anywhere else in the world. The NHS is fundamentally flawed but the system works well for the staff who are employed by it and so doctors, administrators, nurses and politicians are all united in having a vested interest in maintaining the status quo. The only people who would benefit from changing the things that are wrong with our hospitals are patients. And nobody seems to care about them.

And yet the NHS is entrenched in the national psyche as `a good thing', and no politician will dare stand up and point to the fact that the emperor isn't wearing any clothes. Every NHS reorganisation fails because each one misses the point which is that the basic premise upon which the NHS was founded (that the existence of the NHS would pretty well eradicate illness) was utterly false.

And so, the politicians and the bureaucrats constantly tinker. Reforming the NHS is like shifting the deckchairs on the Titanic. The names of the organisations, and the inevitable flow charts which describe their relationships, will change but in principle nothing will alter. There will be more administrators. Any who are made redundant will be given absurdly over-generous severance payments and rehired almost immediately on better terms.

Changes to the NHS are always made for financial and management and political reasons; they are never made for medical reasons. Changes are made to suit the politicians and the administrators. Changes are never made because they will make things better for patients. The patient has long since been forgotten, a bloody nuisance to be brushed to one side whenever decisions are made. The NHS has always been an unfriendly monster and patients have always struggled to cope. In any bureaucracy, doing nothing is always the best and safest option. And opposing *real* change is always a good career move. The NHS is constantly being reorganised but none of the reorganisations affects the big issues. This is no accident. The bureaucrats never change anything important because they know that real change would reduce their power and displease their masters: the politicians and the drug company bosses.

29. How Sensible Living Is Penalised

The NHS encourages people to ignore their own health. Those who smoke, indulge in all the foods that are known to be bad, and allow themselves to become obscenely overweight are, as much as possible, protected from the consequences. The NHS takes all the authority and responsibility away from people. People now believe that if they fall ill then it is someone else's responsibility to make them well again. The healthy, those who do look after their health, end up subsidising the careless and deliberately incautious. Millions now think only of their rights and entitlements; they expect the system to look after them whatever happens.

The heavy drinking, heavy smoking, heroin using, over-weight, promiscuous homosexual man who never uses condoms and who has a penchant for motor car racing and hang-gliding will probably have to pay over the odds for his life insurance. The underwriters know that his chances of living long enough to enable them to make a profit out of an ordinary premium are pretty slim.

Similarly, the driver who is involved in a road accident and who is shown afterwards to have had far too much to drink, to have driven on bald tyres and to have left his seat belt dangling on its hook could find that his chances of getting massive damages are low.

This link between behaviour and consequence encourages people to be careful, to think for themselves and to assess the odds before behaving rashly.

But one disastrous consequence of the NHS is that it diminishes any sense of personal responsibility by separating behaviour from consequences.

And because there is always going to be a shortage of medical equipment and medical personnel, and because the NHS must therefore ration health care, those who are ill through no fault of their own will often suffer because of the deliberate, selfish stupidity of others.

People who recklessly play `catch me if you can' with cancer by eating meat or smoking cigarettes are creating longer waiting lists for everyone. Many careful, sensible individuals die because of the rank stupidity of smokers, heavy drinkers and over-eaters.

Nearly 40 years ago I wrote an article pointing out that I could see nothing wrong with making people pay for their own contrariness. Since it has been established beyond reasonable doubt that many of those who need medical help have knowingly and recklessly damaged their own health, why should the rest of us be prepared to pay for their medical care? Why should the man who regularly smokes 30 cigarettes a day expect the nation to pay for treatment for his bronchitis, his lung cancer, his heart disease and his gastritis? Why should the woman who refuses to diet expect others to help pay when her obesity causes medical problems? Why should the man who persists in drinking too much get free treatment when his liver finally fails to cope? Why should the meat eater expect to receive free medical care when he or she develops colon cancer, breast cancer, prostate cancer, endometrial cancer, rectal cancer, pancreatic cancer or kidney cancer? There is, after all, plenty of research available proving that those cancers are linked to eating meat.

The Health Service is so desperately short of funds, equipment and staff that every year thousands of people who need treatment, and who could be saved, are left to die. Many thousands more die before they can be properly investigated because hospital departments and hospital beds are filled with patients who have only themselves to blame for their ill health.

Why should those idiots who have deliberately exposed themselves to disease receive free care while others, less selfish and more sensible, are left untreated? Why should the drunken driver have his injuries treated free of charge? Why should the climber who sets off in bad weather expect the nation to pay the cost of his rescue and subsequent treatment? These people should pay for the treatment they need. They should take responsibility for their own actions instead of expecting the State to take on that responsibility. Without this proper allocation of responsibility all our freedoms will continue to be diminished. If people knew that they would have to pay for medical treatment for conditions caused or exacerbated by their own stupidity, many would suddenly find that they could give up smoking, give up drinking, give up eating meat, go on a diet, afford new tyres or get back from the pub without using the car.

But the enthusiastic supporters of the NHS cannot bear to think of there being any overt attempt to encourage sensible behaviour. And so we continue to have a system which discourages personal responsibility and diminishes the value of preventive medicine. Too many people rush to the doctor for advice because it is all free. Too few realise that treatment can sometimes be damaging. If there was even a small financial incentive to look after themselves people would be much more careful. The attitude of many is: `I have made myself ill. It's your fault. You should have stopped me. Now it's your job to give me pills and make me better'. Maybe Bevan should have introduced some sort of no-claims bonus system into his blueprint for the NHS.

30. Needless Cuts

At least a quarter of all surgical operations performed are unnecessary.

For some types of surgery - for example: heart surgery, tonsillectomies, circumcisions, caesarian sections for pregnant women and hysterectomies - the percentage of unnecessary operations is almost certainly much higher. At least 90% of all heart surgery is unnecessary. With many operations (such as hernia repair) the downside is often considerably greater than the upside.

Operations are done unnecessarily for a huge variety of reasons. Some - particularly those performed on private patients - may be done because the surgeon needs the cash. Some patients are put down on the list for surgery in order to keep waiting lists long - so that more patients are prepared to pay for private treatment. And some unnecessary operations are done because it's easier to cut open a patient than it is to think about alternatives. If you go to a Ford garage the salesman will recommend a Ford motor car. If you visit a surgeon he will recommend surgery.

As the surplus of doctors continues to grow so the number of unnecessary operations continues to increase. And it isn't just a problem because of the unnecessary pain and discomfort that patients have to put up with. At least 1% of the patients who undergo surgery will die on the operating table or in the ward afterwards. One in every 100 patients who goes into hospital for an operation does not walk out again afterwards.

Of course, some patients are very ill when they are wheeled into the operating theatre.

And some patients would have died without surgery.

But many patients are perfectly healthy when they are taken into the operating theatre. They are having surgery because they have been persuaded by doctors that it is necessary, or that it will in some way improve the quality of their lives.

Back in 1988 (in a book called *The Health Scandal*) I reported that coronary artery bypass surgery (the commonest procedure performed in cardiac surgery) had been in use for nearly 30 years without anyone trying to find out how patients' everyday lives were affected by the operation. When a survey was eventually done it was found that whereas nearly half of the patients who had the operation had been working right up to the time of surgery, three months after the operation only just over a third of the men were working. And a year after the operation nearly half of the patients were still not working. In other words, the operation had little positive effect on patients' lives but did put a good many out of action for some time. And there were, of course, a number of patients who died as a result of surgical complications. A bypass operation takes several hours to perform, consumes a good deal of hospital time and professional skill and can be a physically and mentally exhausting experience for a patient and his family. There is a one in 30 risk that a patient undergoing coronary artery bypass surgery will be dead within 30 days of the operation. The mortality rate varies from surgeon to surgeon but it can be as high as 20% and anything up to a quarter of patients having the operation have heart attacks either while on the operating table or shortly afterwards.

And what makes the medical profession's enthusiasm for coronary artery surgery even more bizarre is the fact that patients who have symptoms of heart disease don't need surgery at all, but stand a better chance of recovering if they are put on a regime which includes a vegan diet, gentle exercise and relaxation. (I described the utterly convincing evidence for this in my book *How To Stop Your Doctor Killing You*, which was first published in 1996. The chapter is entitled *Conquer Heart Disease Without Pills Or Surgery*.)

I can understand cardiac surgeons promoting heart surgery - it is for them a major source of income - but what the hell are GPs doing still referring patients for heart surgery? Any GP who does so should be struck off the medical register and have his stethoscope stuffed up a suitably ill-designed orifice.

31. Doctors Bought: Lock, Stock And Syringe Barrel

Enthusiasm for vaccination has became almost hysterical in much of the world. Drug companies promote vaccination programmes because they make billions of dollars out of vaccines. Doctors are equally enthusiastic because they can charge huge fees for vaccinating their patients. And Governments everywhere are enthusiastic because they have been told (by drug companies and doctors) that vaccination programmes help prevent disease and therefore save money.

But the enthusiasm for vaccination is, in my considered view, a massive confidence trick. There is now much talk in America and Europe of compulsory vaccination programmes being introduced. It is one of the great scandals of our time that doctors promote vaccination with such enthusiasm when vaccines aren't safe and don't work very well. But then, in their defence, they do get paid very well for promoting vaccination. There are already doctors who recommend that *all* children should be vaccinated, whether or not their parents approve. It is likely that those parents who refuse to have their children vaccinated will have them taken away from them. As Dr Ron Paul, former American Presidential Candidate, has pointed out: `When we give Government the power to make medical decisions for us, we, in essence, accept that the State owns our bodies.'

Compulsory vaccinations have already been introduced in some areas of the world and in Britain some GPs (family doctors) are already refusing to look after patients if they don't agree to have their children vaccinated. (There is a financial reason for this. If patients refuse vaccination, British family doctors lose out on huge cash bonuses.)

I now have no doubt that despite the dangers and inefficiencies known to be associated with it, vaccination will become compulsory in the West. The hazards and inadequacies will be ignored. It will not be the first time. Compulsory vaccination was introduced in Britain in the mid 19th century and in 1871 Public Vaccinators were appointed.

There are already many senior members of the medical establishment in Europe and America who want vaccination to be compulsory. You will not be convulsed with shock when I tell you that drug companies which make vaccines would not be averse to their products being made compulsory. I understand that. I would like my books to be made compulsory reading.

The French have already started talking about mass vaccination programmes. I have absolutely no doubt that compulsory vaccination is EU policy. And since the EU always gets what it wants, compulsory vaccination will come to be.

One local authority in England has already created secret vaccination centres, stating that it is doing so under `special powers granted to HM Government under the Civil Contingencies Act 2004'.

Senior doctors recently suggested not only that vaccination should be compulsory but that children who were not vaccinated should not be allowed into school. Social workers will be quick (and eager) to take children away from parents who oppose vaccination.

Politicians have been persuaded that vaccinating the population at large helps save money. The theory is that if you vaccinate 1,000,000 children against, say, whooping cough and, as a result, you prevent 1,000 children getting the disease then the country will avoid the cost of 1,000 parents staying at home for a week or so to look after their child. If one child is permanently brain damaged by the vaccine that is bad luck on the child and his or her parents but, as long as the State can avoid financial responsibility by denying that there is any link between vaccination and brain damage, then it is ahead of the game. In reality, the evidence shows that even this cold-blooded, steel-hearted philosophy is faulty. The problem is that vaccines are so ineffective and so dangerous that instead of being an advantage to society as a whole they are a costly disadvantage.

Drug companies make huge amounts of money out of selling vaccines. And the establishment has fiddled the evidence, and denied or suppressed the inconvenient truths, in order to promote the official point of view. In Britain I have been banned from speaking to doctors. Debates about vaccination are unknown.

The global vaccine market reached $21 billion in 2010 and is growing at a rate of 16.5%. The whole business of vaccinating people is so hugely profitable (largely because it is something that doesn't rely on finding a large number of sick people but also because it is something that can be done on a regular basis) that drug companies, having almost saturated the `vaccinating-children' market are moving heavily into adult vaccines. There is, for example, a vaccine planned to prevent atherosclerosis. I suspect that doctors will claim that this will enable people to keep eating a bad diet and yet avoid heart attacks.

Those who promote vaccines often claim that vaccination programmes have reduced illness, prevented millions of deaths and are the main reason why the average life expectation has risen.

These are all barefaced lies.

The whole vaccination story is one of the great modern scandals of our time. The entire medical profession (at least the part of it in general practice) has been bribed by the drug industry, working through the Government and using taxpayers' money.

The few doctors who do stand up and say something, and who dare to point out that vaccination programmes are a hazard and do more harm than good, tend to be quickly silenced. They are discredited and scorned and their work is not published.

The truth is that most doctors, whether working as hospital consultants, GPs or public health officials, know very little about vaccination. The majority simply follow the establishment line, never question what they are told by the drug industry and dismiss all critics of vaccination as dangerous lunatics.

I do not intend to repeat all the evidence here (it is available in books of mine, including *Superbody*, *Coleman's Laws* and *Animal Experiments Simple Truths* and on my website www.vernoncoleman.com). My book *Anyone Who Tells You Vaccines Are Safe And Effective Is Lying. Here's The Proof* is packed with information about vaccination.

In Britain, doctors give a number of vaccines to babies with developing immune systems. They start dumping the damned stuff into babies when they are two-months-old, for heaven's sake. And yet there is no evidence that vaccines are safe in the long-term. No research is done to check this. The establishment puts the onus on the doubters to find the evidence, knowing that is pretty well impossible. In the USA, a huge medical practice of paediatricians with 30,000 child patients do not vaccinate their patients at all. Guess how many patients with autism they have? If you guessed `none' you guessed right.

In Britain, politicians, doctors, nurses and journalists all enthusiastically insist that vaccines are entirely safe and free from side effects. They are all lying. Lest you assume that is hyperbole let me point out that when, in April 2011, the US Health Department's National Vaccine Injury Compensation Programme released its figures for 2010 the report showed that allegedly safe childhood vaccines officially killed or injured no less than 2,699 children in the year 2010 in America. And the American Government is reported to have also paid out damages to the parents of children with autism - accepting that vaccines can cause autism. In 2010 alone the parents of vaccine damaged children received $110 million in damages from the American Government. Can you imagine the fuss there would be if a food company marketed a product which killed or injured 2,699 healthy children in a single year?

The evidence shows that vaccination programmes have not done the things they are credited with but have done most of the things they are blamed for. The decline in disease, the reduction in infant mortality rates and the increase in average life expectation are all due to improved living conditions. Cleaner water, efficient methods of removing sewage, fresher food, less poverty and less overcrowding are the real reasons why these improvements have taken place. Anyone who doubts this has only to look at graphs showing mortality rates and life expectation rates alongside graphs showing when vaccines were introduced. The graphs show clearly that the improvements took place *before* vaccines were introduced.

Why don't doctors say anything?

Sadly, that is because the medical profession has been bought. GPs lost their final scrap of integrity on the day when they agreed to take money if they managed to vaccinate enough patients. That sort of conveyor belt, bonus-ridden philosophy is better suited to the manufacture of motor car parts than the practise of medicine.

In Britain, GPs receive huge bonus payments if they vaccinate enough patients. Every vaccination they give (or authorise) is another nice noise in the cash register. Epidemics produce a bonus. The Government and the enormous and rich vaccine industry have bought the medical profession, lock stock and syringe barrel. GPs, once members of a proud and distinguished profession which gave us such medical giants as Joseph Lister, have been reduced to snivelling, whining needle-men for the drug industry; hand-maidens to an industry which cares nothing for people but everything for profits. Doctors have lost their way. GPs who jab enough patients receive a thumping great wodge of cash. Any GP who is questioning and discerning will be punished. And so the vast majority of GPs do as they are told. Most know nothing about the dangers of the damned vaccines they so happily jab into patients' arms. Question the whole damned sordid business and these ill-educated propagandists (who know nothing about the risks of the toxic mixtures they are promoting) will throw up their hands in horror. Ask them for some evidence that vaccines are safe and effective and they become hysterical. Facts are, as John Adams said, stubborn things. And the facts do not show any value in vaccination.

Most Western doctors long ago lost any sense of right or wrong. They long ago lost the passions and beliefs and yearnings that (hopefully) took them into medicine. Today, the lives of the vast majority of practising doctors are driven by a potent and destructive (and distinctly patient-unfriendly) mixture of ambition, greed and denial. There are very few Western doctors in practice today who want to save the world, or even change it very much. Their aims are selfish and personal. A bigger house, a faster car, shorter working hours and longer holidays.

As a result, the number of health problems (varying from autism to severe brain damage) caused by vaccines is soaring. The link between vaccinations and illness will continue to be as strenuously denied as was the link between smoking and lung cancer but countries which have not yet adopted mass vaccination programmes would, perhaps, be wise to ask some serious questions before starting to do so.

Just about every healthy individual in the 'developed' world will at some time or another be vaccinated. Individuals who have absolutely nothing wrong with them visit their doctor and allow themselves to be vaccinated in the belief that they are being injected with something perfectly safe which will protect them from disease in the future.

Sadly, there is now a dramatic amount of evidence to show that their faith is misplaced and that vaccines may cause an enormous amount of trouble - and do serious and possibly irreparable harm.

Most practising doctors and nurses at the sharp end of medicine undoubtedly believe that vaccines have helped wipe out some of the deadliest infectious diseases. Many members of the medical profession would put vaccination high on any list of great medical discoveries. The mythical power of vaccination programmes has for years constantly been sustained by Governments and organisations such as the World Health Organisation announcing that such and such a disease will be eradicated when the relevant vaccination programme has been completed.

The theory is that when an individual is given a vaccine - which consists of a weakened or dead version of the disease against which protection is required - his or her body will be tricked into developing antibodies to the disease in exactly the same way that a body develops antibodies when it is exposed to the disease itself.

But in reality things aren't quite so simple. How long do the antibodies last? Do they always work? What about those individuals who don't produce antibodies at all? Vaccination, like so much of western medicine, is a far more inexact science than doctors (and drug companies) would like us to think.

Vaccination is widely respected by doctors and others in the health care industry because of the assumption that it is through vaccination that many of the world's most lethal infectious diseases have been eradicated. But the introduction of vaccination programmes came when the death rates from the major infectious diseases had already fallen. There isn't any evidence to show that vaccination programmes have ever been any of any real value - either to individuals or to communities. When you study (as I have) the evidence relating to whooping cough, tetanus, diphtheria and other diseases it is clear that the incidence, and number of deaths were in decline long before the relevant vaccines were introduced. But as the years have gone by the number of vaccines available has increased steadily. Modern American children receive around 30 vaccinations by the time they go to school. A decade or two ago the only vaccines available were against a relatively small number of diseases including smallpox, tuberculosis, polio, cholera, diphtheria, tetanus and whooping cough. Today, the number of available vaccines seems to grow almost daily. In the past vaccines were produced against major killer diseases. Today, vaccines are produced against diseases such as measles, mumps and chickenpox which have been traditionally regarded as relatively benign inconveniences of childhood.

Does anyone know what happens inside the body when all these different vaccinations are given together? Do different vaccines work with or against one another? What about the risk of interactions? Exactly how does the immune system cope when it is suddenly bombarded with so much foreign material?

Tragically, many doctors seem to know very little about the vaccines they advocate. In my view, if a doctor wants to vaccinate you or a member of your family you should insist that he confirm in writing that the vaccine is both entirely safe and absolutely essential. You may notice his enthusiasm for the vaccine suddenly diminish.

Why are so many people still enthusiastic about vaccination? Well, I suspect that could be because most people simply don't know the truth. The reality is that the truth, regarded as inconvenient, is frequently suppressed. The same thing happens everywhere these days. When I wrote a short-lived column for a newspaper in China the editors were at first reluctant to publish a column I had written criticising vaccination. Eventually, the editors published the piece (simply because I refused to provide an alternative). After the column appeared, my book publishers in China wrote to tell me that the Chinese Government had informed them that they could no longer publish my books. My publishers in China had produced four of my books, all of which had sold very well, but they had been told by the Government that only `medical publishing houses' could in future publish books concerned with health care. Other Chinese publishers who had shown great enthusiasm for publishing my books also suddenly changed their minds.

32. How And Why Doctors Ignore The Major Cause Of Illness

There is clear medical and scientific evidence available to show that nothing, not even tobacco, influences your chances of developing cancer as much as the food you choose to eat. It is estimated that between 30% and 60% of all cancers are caused by what you eat. Doctors, scientists and supporters of the cancer industry (all of whom realise that there is no money to be made out of preventing cancer, but tons of loot to be made out of doing research and flogging `cures' and treatments) merrily ignore this fact and claim that the battle against cancer will only be won with the aid of more money. They claim that in order to obtain the information we need we must spend, spend, spend. But that isn't true. It is not more knowledge we need (we have, as I pointed out in *Paper Doctors* nearly 40 years ago, already amassed far more knowledge than we will ever use in our lifetime), but the ability and courage and determination to use the knowledge we already have. And the evidence proving that certain types of food cause cancer has been available for a remarkably long time.

Amazingly, it has for many years been widely agreed that 80% of all cancers are preventable - using knowledge which we have available at the moment. In other words ignorance (sustained through political and industrial expediency) is responsible for 80% of the millions of deaths caused by cancer each year. And much of that ignorance involves the effect that food has upon the health.

Way back in 1981, it was estimated that dietary modifications might result in a one third reduction in the number of deaths from cancer in the United States with a 90% reduction in deaths from cancer of the stomach and large bowel; a 50% reduction in deaths from cancers of the endometrium, gallbladder, pancreas and breast; a 20% reduction in deaths from cancers of the lung, larynx, bladder, cervix, mouth, pharynx and oesophagus and a 10% reduction in deaths from other sites.

Back in 1982, the National Research Council in the United States of America published a technical report entitled *Diet, Nutrition and Cancer* which showed that diet was probably the single most important factor in the development of cancer, and, even then, 30 years ago, that there was evidence linking cancers of the breast, colon and prostate to particular foods or types of food.

It is a scandal of astonishing proportions that a majority of the population still do not know about these vitally important and well-established links. It is an even bigger scandal that most doctors still dismiss the idea of a food/cancer link as mumbo-jumbo nonsense, preferring to rely entirely on prescription drugs, radiotherapy and surgery as `treatments' for cancer. The average medical student probably spends more time staring down a microscope at histology slides than he or she spends studying nutrition.

Today, it is an undeniable fact that between a third and a half of all cancers are caused by eating the wrong types of food and you can dramatically reduce your chances of developing cancer of the breast, cancer of the prostate, cancer of the colon, cancer of the ovary or cancer of the uterus by not eating meat. And yet when I checked one large (over 1,000 pages long) medical textbook I found that the chapter on cancer summed up the role of food as a causal agent in just one, rather short, sentence. I find this all extremely difficult to understand. I have been studying scientific research papers for over four decades and I have never seen such convincing research as that which shows the links between particular types of food and particular types of cancer. I have absolutely no doubt that if these undeniable links had been properly publicised countless millions of lives could - and would - have been saved. The suppression of this information by a greedy and conscience-free food industry, compliant, revenue conscious politicians, a cancer industry dominated by grant-hungry researchers and an uncaring, drug company dominated medical profession has, I sincerely believe, led to more deaths than any war in history.

Since the early 1980s the amount of evidence linking diet to cancer has grown steadily. In 1990 even the British Medical Association, hardly an organisation which would be widely described as revolutionary, supported the view that there is a link between food and cancer. Their published view was that 35% of cancers are caused by the natural constituents of food and that another 1 per cent of cancers are caused by food additives.

Other organisations suggest that the link between food and cancer is even higher. The National Academy of Sciences in the United States, founded in 1863 by Act of Congress to serve as an official adviser to the US Government in all matters of science and technology, has reported that researchers have estimated that almost 60% of women's cancers and a little more than 40% of men's cancers are related to nutritional factors. (Readers who want to see more evidence proving that meat causes cancer will find it on my website www.vernoncoleman.com.)

The evidence linking meat eating to illness and death is incontestable. Meat eaters have three times the risk of developing diabetes, compared with vegans. Red and processed meats are clearly linked to colon cancer and other forms of the disease. And of course meat products are often contaminated with faecal bacteria, leading to deadly infections. (Meat products may include bits of chopped up animal cancer as well as animal bowels - complete with the faeces inside.) Consumption of red and processed meats increases the risks of bladder cancer. A study of over 300,000 men and women found that those who consumed the most red meat had a 22% increased risk of bladder cancer, compared with those who ate the least. Consumption of nitrites and nitrates (substances used for preserving, colouring and flavouring processed meats) was associated with a 28% to 29% increased risk. The study, in the journal *Cancer* was conducted as part of the *NIH-AARP Diet and Health Study*. And eating meat leads to weight gain. The *American Journal of Clinical Nutrition* published a study involving 373,803 participants in the *European Prospective Investigation into Cancer* study. Those who ate 8.8 ounces of meat per day gained more weight year by year, compared with people who ate less meat or none at all. The researchers concluded that reducing meat consumption may help people avoid weight gain. Girls who eat the most meat products during childhood may have an earlier onset of puberty, increasing their risks of diseases such as cancer, heart disease and osteoporosis. Researchers followed 3,298 girls in Bristol, England and found that 49% of girls who ate more than 12 portions of meat per week started their periods by the age of 12, compared with 35% of girls who ate fewer than four portions of meat per week.

But the medical profession refuses to consider this problem. After reading that a doctor in Suffolk was alleged to be 'prescribing' meat for his patients I sent the following letter to the General Medical Council.

'According to the press today a Dr John Cannon of the Ixworth Surgery near Bury St Edmunds, is alleged to be 'prescribing rump steak and pork chops' to his patients to 'keep them healthy'. Would you please investigate Dr Cannon's alleged activities? There is ample evidence available to show that meat causes cancer. I can (and happily will) provide the GMC with over 20 scientific papers, published in reputable journals (including the International Journal of Cancer, New England Journal of Medicine, Cancer Research, British Journal of Cancer, Cancer, British Medical Journal) showing that eating meat causes cancer. The United States Surgeon General has reported links between meat eating and cancer. I look forward to hearing from you. I suggest that this is a matter of significant public interest and should be attended to without delay. From the newspaper reports I understand that Dr Cannon's alleged activities are being encouraged by the British Meat Nutrition Education Service.'

The story of the doctor who 'prescribes' meat appeared in Britain's national press. The doctor himself appeared on British television. The letter I sent to the GMC was sent to all national newspapers in Britain. None of them reported it.

The GMC's response was:

'We have carefully considered the information you provided and understand your reasons for writing to us. However, we have decided that this is not a matter that justifies action by us. The issue you have mentioned does not appear to have any bearing on Dr Cannon's ability to practise medicine and does not breach our guidance. We are therefore unable to take any further action on your complaint.'

With the GMC closing its eyes it is, perhaps, hardly surprising that if you ask 1,000 doctors to name the commonest cause of cancer in Britain I doubt if more than a handful will know the right answer. It is, therefore, hardly surprising that the incidence of cancer is rising rapidly and is going to continue to rise. The main cause of cancer in Britain today is not the smoking of cigarettes but the eating of meat.

Not surprisingly, doctors (much of whose education is controlled by the pharmaceutical industry and a Government controlled by the pharmaceutical industry) prefer to deal with the problems created by meat eating by prescribing drugs. Drugs are always the treatment of choice these days for a profession which is owned needle, syringe and pen by the pharmaceutical industry.

In January 2011 it was, for example, reported that seven million people in the UK were taking drugs called statins, theoretically to prevent heart attacks. Encouraged by the drug industry, GPs were, at a huge cost to the NHS, prescribing the damned things for everyone with a pulse. I first warned of the serious health problems associated with these drugs in the first edition of my book *How To Stop Your Doctor Killing You* back in 1998. But the unholy trinity which controls the NHS doesn't have much interest in science or uncomfortable facts.

(As an aside, it seems strange to me that doctors seem totally uninterested in the fact that feeding people meat is directly responsible for a number of the world's serious problems. First, animals need to be fed grain and if people stopped eating meat there would be plenty of food to go round. The millions starving to death could be fed. Second, growing all the grain needed to feed animals creates havoc for the environment. For example, it takes a million gallons of water to grow just one acre of corn to feed to cattle. And as the water trickles into streams and rivers it carries with it the remains of the fertilisers the farmers used. The fertiliser chemicals pollute the water we drink (as I reported half a lifetime ago it is impossible to remove the chemicals from our drinking water). The fertiliser also makes algae overgrow in our rivers and as the algae decomposes it uses up oxygen in the water, killing the fish. In America, farmers are responsible for the existence of a 8,000 square mile dead zone below Louisiana and Texas. And, of course the 100 million cows in the USA are all belching out methane - which is much more potent as a greenhouse gas than carbon dioxide. But doctors don't worry about any of this stuff.)

Incidentally, food doesn't just *cause* cancer.

It can help stop you recovering too.

However careful you are to avoid potentially cancerous chemicals, cancer cells will occasionally develop inside your body. Most of the time those cancer cells are dealt with speedily and effectively by your body's defence systems. White blood cells find and destroy cancer cells in just the same way that they find and destroy bacteria.

However, your body's natural immune system (and its ability to deal with cancer) will be damaged if you eat the wrong sort of foods - and will be aided and improved if you eat the right foods! Fatty foods will weaken your immune system and make your body less capable of fighting off those occasional cancer cells. When researchers studied the blood of human volunteers they found that a low fat diet greatly improved the activity of the body's natural killer cells. Amazingly, depressingly, cancer specialists and cancer charity workers still don't seem to understand or accept the importance of a healthy immune system in fighting cancer. (As far as the body's immune system is concerned vegetable fats are just as bad as animal fats. In order to protect yourself against cancer you need to reduce your entire fat consumption - and that includes vegetable oils.)

Vegetarians have more than double the cancer cell destroying capability of non-vegetarians. But this is not entirely due to the low fat content of a vegetarian diet. It is probably also due to the fact that vegetarians consume fewer toxic chemicals and no animal proteins. And vegetarians have another advantage too: the ability of the human body's natural, killer cells to do their work is improved by substances such as beta-carotene which are found in considerable quantities in vegetables. (One survey of meat eaters showed that many could neither name nor describe any green vegetables).

Food provides us with the building blocks we need to grow and to stay alive. If we don't eat the right food we fall ill. If we are ill and don't eat the right food we won't get well. Most people know this. Most people, that is, except the people who work in hospitals. The doctors, the nurses, the cooks, the dieticians and the administrators either don't know or don't care.

The food in hospitals is diabolical and contributes enormously to the death rate among patients. It seems rather crazy to give hospital patients a food item (meat) that is known to cause cancer. Food is as big a cause of cancer as tobacco and meat is the biggest culprit. This is fact, not opinion. Sadly, most nutritionists, dieticians and chefs are woefully ignorant about food. I don't expect chefs to know anything much about food but dieticians and nutritionists who fail to warn patients that eating meat causes cancer are either stupid or ignorant and should be fired and retrained as lavatory attendants. Hospitals which give their patients meat to eat might as well be handing out free cigarettes. It would make as much sense, do less harm to the environment and probably be cheaper.

Not that it is just the meat in the hospital diet that causes problems. The quality of the food served to patients in our hospitals is beyond appalling. You are more likely to contract a food bug in an NHS hospital than just about anywhere else in Britain. What an awful thing it is that NHS hospital food is more likely to make you ill than a hot dog bought from a street vendor's stall.

The way the food is served is a scandal too. The cleaners put down their mops and hand out the food. Naturally, they don't bother to wash their hands. If the patient is physically incapable of eating what's been put before them then the tray is simply taken away. `Not hungry, dear?' says the cleaner, whisking away the tray as the patient grows weaker and weaker from lack of any sort of food. `We're not allowed to feed patients,' one cleaner told me. `I'm here to nurse,' one overweight nurse told me. `I'm not here to feed patients.' I had a suspicion that she was eating up all the leftovers. It is not unknown for patients who are not visited by relatives to starve to death in hospital.

The bottom line is that the food in most NHS hospitals is at best inedible and at worst dangerous. There is rarely enough of it. It is often badly chosen and badly prepared. Patients of all types desperately need good food if they are to have the best chance of recovering. But food-related illnesses are commonplace in hospitals. And nurses are so lazy and disinterested that thousands of patients starve to death because they cannot reach the food that is put in front of them. Just about every dietician, nutritionist and cook working for the NHS should be charged with multiple manslaughter.

When my mother had breast cancer she wisely stopped eating meat and adopted a vegetarian diet. She did not take the tamoxifen tablets the consultant oncologist prescribed. And she refused the radiotherapy they recommended. She beat the cancer with diet.

When she was admitted to hospital with her final illness the staff were told that she was vegetarian. They took no notice. In both Exeter and Budleigh hospitals the staff persisted in offering her meat-based dishes.

When my mother was given a meal of sausages I complained to one of the nurses. I explained that my mother was vegetarian. The nurse told me that my mother could have a Cornish pasty instead of the sausage.

On another occasion, early in her final illness, I was sitting beside my mother's bed when she was brought a meal consisting of cottage pie and boiled potatoes. Her menu slip had been filled in by someone else because she was too confused to do it herself. 'This is cottage pie,' I said to my mother. 'Do you want it?' She thought for a long time. She was becoming demented but knew that there was something wrong. It was clearly a great effort for her. 'I don't eat cottage pie,' she replied at last. 'Why not?' I asked her quietly. 'It's not the sort of thing I eat,' she replied at last. 'I don't eat meat.'

When we did finally persuade the hospital staff to provide vegetarian food they provided very little variety. When I was feeding her pieces of an insipid looking cheese and leek flan she said, with great heart-felt weariness: 'I've had a lot of that.'

The Government, whose advisers know of the relationship between meat consumption and cancer, spends taxpayers' money on promoting the sale and consumption of meat. Thomas Jefferson was perfectly correct when he wrote: `If people let Government decide what foods they eat, and what medicines they take, their bodies will soon be as sorry state as are the souls of those who live under tyranny.' They might just as well promote the smoking of cigarettes. And despite the fact that people who eat lots of burgers are more likely to develop cancer than people who eat a healthier diet (`Eat McCrap, develop McCancer and McDie' might not be a catchy slogan but I offer it without charge), Britain's Department of Health has invited McDonald's, (and other processed food companies) to help write Government policy on obesity and diet related diseases.

33. Benzo Bonanza

Originally introduced specifically to help calm extremely nervous and agitated patients (and for use as anaesthetics) benzodiazepines were, by the time they reached their peak, being prescribed for just about every illness known to man or woman. When I was campaigning against their over-use in the 1970s and 1980s, I met people who had been prescribed them as treatments for backache, menopausal problems, pre-menstrual tension, migraine, high blood pressure, alopecia and urinary tract infections. It got to the point where doctors were handing out prescriptions for benzodiazepine tranquillisers whenever they didn't know what else to do. There was never any evidence to show that drugs were effective in treating all these different conditions.

As a result, it was hardly surprising that in the UK alone three million people became addicted to these drugs. Benzodiazepine addiction was, and probably still is, the world's biggest drug addiction problem. Governments spend billions on wretched and pointless 'drugs wars' while drug companies are allowed to sell and promote drugs which are far more addictive than heroin, cocaine or cannabis.

Over 30 years ago, I started a campaign to warn patients of the hazards of taking benzodiazepine tranquillisers such as Valium. I felt that the basic problem with tranquillisers was not that patients were addicted to taking them but that doctors were addicted to prescribing the damned things. Way back in the 1988, after a lengthy campaign, I personally persuaded the Government to change the prescribing rules relating to tranquillisers. But doctors *still* over-prescribe these drugs because they are convenient. In the same way that parents stick their children in front of the television set, so doctors prescribe tranquillisers for nervous, time-consuming patients. The television set and the tranquillisers are used for the same reason: to shut people up.

In 1988 the Government, having admitted that it was responding to my books and articles, advised GPs that benzodiazepines should not be prescribed for patients for longer than two to four weeks but in May 2011 it was revealed that 11.5 million prescriptions a year were still being written for benzodiazepine tranquillisers. Over a third of those prescriptions were for more than eight weeks supply. What a bloody profession.

Any doctor who signs a prescription for a benzodiazepine (such as Valium) for more than two weeks is not fit to practise medicine and would, if the General Medical Council did what it is supposed to do, be struck off the medical register. It annoys me immensely that patients who have become addicted to these wretched drugs should be ignored by the NHS whereas whingeing idiots who take drugs such as heroin and cocaine for entertainment are, when they moan about their inevitable condition and demand treatment, instantly provided with vast amounts of support. For the record, benzodiazepines are considerably more addictive than any of the so-called recreational drugs.

34. When A Vegetarian Sausage Beats An MRI Scanner

In the dark old days of medicine, objective judgements were made based on a skilful and knowledgeable interpretation and assessment of a mixture of symptoms and signs. Doctors made diagnoses relying on their own senses, rather than bowing to extremely fallible machines. They relied on experience, instinct and intuition. They used X-rays and laboratory tests to help them confirm their diagnoses.

Today, diagnostic skills are disappearing and doctors are coming to rely almost entirely on laboratory tests and X-ray pictures. Doctors don't dare make diagnoses unless they can provide bits of paper from a laboratory to substantiate their conclusion. Since laboratory tests and investigations are woefully inaccurate, and often misleading, the result is that many patients are wrongly diagnosed (and exposed to unnecessary treatments), many serious problems are missed completely and doctors are making more mistakes than ever.

A growing majority of doctors now do little more than interpret laboratory results; they know that ordering tests is easier than thinking and that they are not likely to be sued if they have bits of paper to support their diagnoses. Doctors have become little more than simple computers: ordering tests and making decisions on the basis of the results obtained. When my wife was taken ill with neurological problems she saw several doctors before anyone thought to ask her about her diet. Numerous tests were performed but no one bothered to ask her what sort of foods she ate. And yet diet is a vital factor in the development of illness.

Modern doctors rely far too much on technology - and far too little on building up any diagnostic skills of their own. Old-fashioned doctors used to rely on what their patients told them and on what their eyes, ears, noses and fingertips told them. Most important of all, perhaps, was the sixth sense that doctors used to acquire through years of clinical experience. Modern doctors rely too much upon equipment which is often faulty, frequently badly calibrated and more often than not downright misleading.

Sadly, doctors seem surprisingly unaware that the high technology alternatives to genuine diagnostic skills are dangerously fallible; they do not seem to know that if you do enough tests you will always find an abnormality. Then the abnormality (which may be entirely harmless) will have to be further investigated and probably treated. Tests are often inaccurate and frequently misleading. They lead to many mistaken diagnoses. (There is a chapter in my book *Coleman's Laws* dealing with the problems created by misleading tests and investigations.) Many doctors seem quite unable, or unwilling, to reach a diagnosis unless the diagnosis is more or less written out on a form that has been printed by a computer. The best diagnostician I ever knew was not a hospital consultant but a GP. He was old and frail when I knew him. He could make diagnoses more accurately than any doctor relying on technology. His secret was simple: he listened to patients and considered their responses; he looked at them and he noticed things. It wasn't complicated. Today's doctors have lost the skill that was most valued among doctors a generation ago: the skill to make diagnoses. (Treating patients who have been diagnosed is, by comparison, straightforward and simple enough. Any fool can open a textbook, look up a disease, and find out how to treat it.) Doctors don't seem to have realised that you don't need six years of medical school to order a pile of laboratory tests. And you don't need six years of training to `read' the results. If doctors are going to continue to rely exclusively on test results when making diagnoses then medical training could be cut down to a weekend.

The X-rays, blood tests and other investigations which doctors order are not just sometimes lethal but are frequently unnecessary. Many tests are wildly inaccurate and dangerously misleading as well. Tests results are often wrong. It is not unusual to obtain 30% false negatives or false positives. This means that if a doctor performs ten tests then the chances are that three of them will be wrong and quite misleading.

Here are just some of the frightening facts that I can reveal about medical investigations:

1. X-rays are the third biggest cause of cancer (after eating meat and smoking). Many X-rays are done quite unnecessarily - just as a 'routine'. In Britain around 20,000 people a year get cancer from medical and dental X-rays. X-rays given to pregnant women during the 1950s and 1960s are responsible for between 5% and 10% of all childhood cancers. Children who develop leukaemia - and other cancers - may have been made ill because their mothers had X-rays while they were pregnant.

2. Tests often wrongly show up disease in healthy individuals. Those patients are then subjected to surgery and drug therapy which they do not need.

3. Tests - which patients and doctors seem to trust too much - often wrongly say that a patient is healthy.

4. About two thirds of all medical tests are worthless and of no help to the patient.

5. Patients routinely admitted to hospital are often subjected to 20 or so blood, urine and other tests. When so many tests are done one or more abnormalities will be found in two thirds of all healthy individuals. Once an abnormal result has been obtained doctors feel obliged to continue doing tests. The tests they do often produce serious complications. Many patients who think they are ill - and

have been told that they need to take drugs for life - are not really ill at all.

6. Unnecessary tests are often done out of habit, for personal research, to provide protection in case of lawsuits or simply to impress other doctors. Doctors frequently order tests because it is quicker and easier to fill in a form than it is to talk and listen or to examine a patient properly.

7. When blood tests are done the results are compared against `normal' values. But the `normal' figures may have been produced decades earlier - by testing a few seemingly healthy doctors and nurses. No one really knows what is `normal'. Your `abnormal' result may be more `normal' than the official `normal' result.

8. Doctors who know that tests can be misleading frequently order expensive, uncomfortable and even hazardous investigations - and then ignore the results.

9. Complicated, expensive and potentially dangerous tests are often ordered when simple, inexpensive and perfectly safe tests would be more appropriate. My wife saw a neurologist who decided that her symptoms might be caused by a tumour affecting the top of her spine. The doctor ordered an MRI scan of her brain and spine. But the disease the doctor had thought possible causes a very specific loss of sensation - including a loss of temperature sensation. I took a frozen vegetarian sausage out of the freezer and performed a simple test myself - using the frozen sausage to check for temperature sensation loss. There were no temperature sensation losses. I concluded that the diagnosis was wrong and we cooked the sausage and ate it. Four days later my wife went for the MRI scan as arranged. The scan supported the evidence provided by the cold vegetarian sausage and showed that there was no lesion in my wife's spine. The sausage test, just as reliable as the scan, took a fraction of the time to do and cost about Ł10,000 less. The results were available instantly.

35. Committees And Quangos

I don't have faith in the medical establishment and I don't have much faith in the advisory committees who give advice on health and food matters to our political leaders and to civil servants.

It is difficult to trust the conclusions and recommendations of official Government committees or quangos because they are, inevitably, peopled by individuals who have been selected because they are compliant rather than complaining. Dissenters don't get picked to sit on committees to advise the Department of Health or the Department of Agriculture. On the contrary, many of the people who give out official guidelines on food and drugs are linked in some way with the food and drug industries - and may, therefore, benefit financially from their own decisions. Under those circumstances it isn't always easy to be certain that our politicians are acting on entirely impartial advice. The evidence of what these people have done in the last few decades could certainly not be used in their defence.

It's the same almost everywhere in the world. Most Government committees consist predominantly of individuals who work for or with the appropriate industries. An American newspaper, *USA Today*, expressed surprise that 54% of 300 experts, sitting on 18 advisory committees, and hired to advise the American Government on the safety and effectiveness of medicines, had a direct financial interest in the drug or subject they were being asked to evaluate. Some of the experts received consulting fees, others had research grants from the companies they were supposed to be investigating and others had shares or stock options. Federal law prohibits the Food and Drug Administration in the USA from using experts with financial conflicts but this law is frequently waived. (It has been waived more than 800 times since 1998).

None of this is anything new, of course. I found worse figures in the UK 20 or 30 years ago (though no British newspaper had the courage to print the findings). Most of the people selected to sit on health committees and quangos work for (or are associated with or have worked for) drug companies. Most of the people selected to sit on food advisory committees work for (or are associated with or have worked for) food companies. Most of the people making decisions about genetic engineering work for (or are associated with or have worked for) the genetic engineering industry.

It is because our bureaucracies are controlled in this way that we end up with absurd regulations which are, it is claimed, intended to protect the consumer but which, in reality, favour industry and do nothing for the consumers.

We have treaties which result in food surpluses being dumped. We have regulations which make it nigh on impossible for people to sell safe, effective remedies which might compete with drug company products. We have regulations requiring food companies to put additives and other chemicals into otherwise edible foods. We have monopolies and genetic engineering hazards everywhere we look.

Global corporations, mostly American, now *own* many of the seeds of established crops. An American company has been given a patent in basmati rice. The peasants who perfected this variety of rice now cannot use it unless they pay the company holding the patent. Peasants can no longer sow the seeds they save from the plants they grow. They must buy their seeds, every year, from big American seed companies. The peasants can't afford to do this. So the poor people in countries around the world starve to death. Governments and charities have to intervene, and use your money and my money, to keep people alive and, in doing so, help ensure the continued, rising profits of these companies.

A generation ago the average dairy cow produced eight quarts of milk a day. Today, a typical cow produces 50 quarts a day. Just how do you think the farmers have changed nature so dramatically? Why haven't any Government advisors asked questions? A generation ago cows ate grass. Today cows are fed blood and bone taken from other cows. Cows are herbivores but farmers feed them bits of other cows, though they do have the decency to wait until the other cows are dead. A generation ago milk was banned if it contained more than a trace of antibiotics. Today milk is stuffed with antibiotics and other drugs. One expert reported finding 52 different residues of antibiotics in a sample of milk in the USA.

The world has gone crazy.

Chickens are fed on a mixed diet of cardboard and animal shit, for heaven's sake.

And it is the so-called independent experts who sit on committees and advise Governments who have allowed all this to happen. It is utterly absurd that so many of the individuals who sit on committees given the responsibility of regulating the products of the drug industry have, or have had, lucrative contracts with drug companies.

Whenever I have confronted politicians with the fact that members of powerful committees have drug company links they have responded by arguing that all doctors have drug company links and so it is impossible to find alternatives. This is patently untrue. The sad truth is that free thinking individuals, who are not beholden to industry, are never likely to find themselves sitting on any of these committees.

36. Medical Screening Is Expensive And Doesn't Work

The principle of screening is a simple one: the patient trots along to the doctor and the doctor (for a chunky great fee, of course) does tests which are designed to spot early signs of cancer or other diseases. But screening doesn't work. It's actually very dangerous. A once-a-year check-up is no alternative to a healthier lifestyle. Doctors are, however, enthusiastic about screening because it's enormously profitable. And they're very lukewarm about encouraging their patients to follow healthier lifestyles because there is no money in it.

In several earlier books I have explained why I neither approve of nor support the principle of medical screening programmes. On balance they do far more harm than good.

For decades now just about every attempt to show that medical screening programmes save lives has proved that they are a waste of time, energy and money. Indeed, surveys have proved that, because of the risk of false positives, medical screening programmes do more harm than good.

Medical screening programmes go back a long way. The first recorded screening took place at a public brothel in Avignon in 1347 when a local Abbess and a surgeon examined all the working women every Saturday to see whether or not they were fit to carry on serving the local population.

Modern screening really started in 1917 in the U.S. when large corporations thought it might be a good idea to have their employees examined regularly. When half of four million American men called up for military service during the first World War proved to be unfit for military service insurance companies started screening the general population.

Since then the medical screening business has grown virtually unchecked - despite the fact that since the 1970s there has been ample evidence to show that medical screening programmes are not just a waste of time and money but can also be a serious health hazard.

Over 30 years ago, in 1979, the World Health Organisation published a report which showed that people who were subjected to regular medical screenings needed to go to hospital more often but were not as healthy as people who did not undergo regular medical screenings. The conclusion was that health screening is expensive and ineffective.

In the same year (1979) the results of a Canadian Task Force report on Periodic Health Examination came to the conclusion that annual medical check-ups should be abandoned since they are both inefficient and potentially harmful.

Those who have studied general health screening programmes with an open mind have come to the conclusion that they are harmful for four reasons.

First, when people are taught to put their faith in medical check-ups they tend to abandon responsibility for their own health and enjoy a false sense of security. Patients forget that a medical check-up is no more a sign of long-term health than an encouraging bank statement is a sign of permanent financial security. A patient who is given a clean bill of health is likely to ignore strange symptoms which develop a week or two later. And there is a danger that he (or she) may feel that it is unnecessary to eat wisely or to take regular exercise.

Second, screening examinations may frighten people. They can result in cancer phobias, neuroses and depression. And they can result in so much stress that the immune system is damaged - leading to a greater susceptibility to disease.

Third, the procedures involved in screening programmes may do physical harm. There are, for example, some doctors who perform coronary angiographs as part of their check-up procedures. As many as two patients per 100 may die during this procedure.

Fourth, when a screening examination results in a false positive the patient may be given a treatment which may damage his or health. A major Swedish report on breast screening showed that out of 600,000 women screened there had been 100,000 false positives.

When specific screening programmes are studied, more evidence of their lack of value becomes evident. For example, cervical screening programmes have been popular for decades. And they are often held up as an example of just how useful screening programmes can be. But cervical screening programmes are as pointless as they are expensive. Just about every so-called developed country in the world has a cervical screening programme. Naturally, the NHS spends huge amounts of time and effort on cervical screening. But here are a few facts about cervical screening which are not widely known.

First, no one can agree on when or how often cervical smears should be taken. And so programmes tend to be fairly random and haphazard.

Second, no tests have ever been done to find out how cervical screening should be done. The smear test is neither accurate nor reliable. Doctors frequently take smears from the wrong site - or use faulty techniques. Different cytologists reading the same slide may produce entirely different results. Abnormal cells may be present in one sample and not in another from the same woman. The widespread chaos and confusion that exists is a result of simple ignorance.

Third, although vast amounts of public money are spent on cervical screening programmes there is no evidence to show that these programmes have made any difference at all to mortality rates. If cervical screening worked one might reasonably expect the number of women dying from cervical cancer to have fallen since screening was introduced. It hasn't.

Fourth, cervical cancer is, despite all the political hype, a relatively uncommon killer. Even carcinoma of the pancreas kills more women than carcinoma of the cervix. It's a pretty safe bet that if the money wasted on cervical screening programmes had been spent warning women of the dangers of eating meat then thousands of lives would have been saved. I also believe that the mortality rate from cervical cancer would fall if women were encouraged to ask for medical help if they noticed any unusual signs or symptoms - such as bleeding between periods or after intercourse. I can't prove that offering such simple advice would be of value because no one has done any trials or tests to find out whether it would. Why not? Who would make any profit out of offering such simple advice? (In the same way, what profit can there possibly be in teaching women how to examine their own breasts?)

Cervical screening programmes have, over the years, consistently attracted huge budgets. Untold thousands of doctors have been employed in performing cervical smears. The laudable aim of the cervical screening programme has always been to reduce the number of women dying from cervical cancer and it has constantly been argued that if more money were put into cervical screening programmes thousands of lives could be saved.

But I don't think the evidence supports this contention.

Most worrying is the fact that many of the smears taken by doctors are useless. One report concluded that 10% of all cervical smears sent to cytology departments were useless and a further 40% were of limited usefulness in detecting carcinoma of the cervix. The main problems are that doctors either take smears from the wrong site or use faulty techniques. There is, surprisingly perhaps, still a considerable amount of confusion about the natural history of the cervical cancer. From the evidence I've seen it seems possible that some slow growing cancers might regress if left alone while fast growing cancers could develop so rapidly that smears would have to be done every few months to be of real value.

One report concluded that a third of the biopsies performed because of positive cervical cytology were likely to have been performed for lesions which were insignificant or would have disappeared if left alone. Since the biopsies were performed under anaesthetic (with which there is always a risk of death) it seems perfectly possible that for these women the dangers associated with having a smear might have been greater than the possible advantages.

Sadly, even when useful smears are taken the laboratories providing results cannot always cope. And even when laboratories do discover significant changes women are not always notified. Delays mean that at least one woman has died after having had a positive smear but before she had been given her results. And there is, not surprisingly, an enormous amount of confusion among gynaecologists about the best way to treat cervical cancer even when it has been identified.

Indeed, a cynical observer might be inclined to suggest that it is the medical profession which has benefited most from the cervical screening programme. One leading physician described the results of screening for cervical cancer in Britain as `disappointing'. A writer in one leading international journal argued that `there is no clear evidence that this screening is beneficial, and it may well be doing more harm than good'.

Although doctors around the world have strongly argued in favour of more expenditure on smears they have never really decided exactly which women need to be targeted. And there have never been any trials done which show the undisputed value of the cervical screening programme. I don't believe that the cervical screening programme has ever been properly evaluated.

Indeed, the evidence rather suggests that cervical screening programmes may not be of any real value to women as a whole - though there will, of course, always be individual women who are able to say that their lives were `saved'.

Statistically, the test has not been shown to save lives in any country where it has been introduced. Huge amounts of public money have been spent on organised cervical screening programmes but the incidence of cervical cancer has hardly altered in 30 years. In countries where the incidence of cervical cancer and the number of women dying from it are falling the rate of decline is no greater than it was before the screening programme began.

Britain, for example, has spent several billion pounds on its cervical screening programme but the programme has never been based on any logical plan and the number of women dying from cervical cancer has hardly changed. In fact, because the disease is relatively uncommon (cervical cancer does not make the top ten list of causes of death among women), huge numbers of women who do not have the disease have been subjected to unnecessary tests. And because `false positives' are fairly common (women being told that they have cancer when they don't) many women have been referred unnecessarily for further tests and treatment. Even more worryingly `false negatives' occur in between 7% and 60% of smears. And an enormous amount of anxiety and fear are produced by the often inefficient and thoughtless way in which smear reports are submitted to patients. I can't prove it but I suspect that the cervical cancer programme has caused more cancer than it has found.

The enthusiasm of doctors for cervical screening is not difficult to understand. The medical profession's enthusiasm for cervical screening was aroused by, and is sustained by, the profit to be made, rather than any belief that cervical screening will save lives. In one medical journal a writer pointed out that: `unless doctors take urgent individual action a serious breakdown in cervical smear recalls - affecting GP income - could arise in five years' time.'

I believe that if the money spent on doctors' fees had been spent on educational programmes many thousands more lives could have been saved.

Breast screening is today even more fashionable than cervical screening. It is, however, of even more questionable value.

It is well over a quarter of a century since I first warned about the futility of doctor-dependant breast screening programmes (very shortly after these expensive and highly profitable programmes had been being introduced).

In my book *The Health Scandal* (which was published in 1988 and violently attacked by doctors all over the country - even though some of those who were doing the attacking admitted that they hadn't actually bothered to read it) I objected to mammography screening partly on the grounds that I thought there must surely be risks in having regular X-ray examinations (it would, I thought, be hideously, grotesquely ironic if a new technique designed to spot breast cancer at an early stage turned out, 20 years later, to cause breast cancer) and partly on the grounds that a mass breast screening programme simply would not work and would not make a significant difference to the number of women dying of breast cancer because the interval of one year between examinations was too long.

Even before I wrote *The Health Scandal* I was convinced that the potential health hazards which might be associated with mammograms could outweigh the advantages. This conviction was not based on any inside knowledge. It always seemed to me pretty obvious that repeatedly subjecting breast tissue (which is known to be prone to cancer) to X-rays (which is known to cause cancer) could be hazardous. This seems to me to be a fairly obvious concern. But it is one which the medical establishment regularly dismissed as not even worth consideration. (Relatively recent research has, however, shown that one woman in every 1,000 screened will develop breast cancer in the two years following the X-ray.) Moreover, it seemed to me that the risks associated with mammograms should have been properly assessed before mass mammography was introduced. (Why is common sense so uncommon - and so derided by those who consider themselves to be above such things?)

I pointed out that the available evidence showed clearly that self-examination was much better and more effective (as well as being considerably cheaper and requiring far less highly trained medical manpower). `A proper educational programme,' I wrote, `designed to teach British women how to examine their breasts properly, would undoubtedly have a dramatic effect on the number of women dying from breast cancer in Britain. It would cost very little and it would produce continuing results. But it would not, of course, provide work for the many unwanted radiologists who we are training every year. And it probably wouldn't satisfy the strident spokeswomen who believe that annual screening clinics must be better than regular checks done at home.'

At the time this comment was dismissed as heresy by many in the medical establishment who argued that self-screening was useless. But, gradually, more doctors began to question the logic of mammography. And then several studies suggested that the radiation accumulated through yearly mammograms might actually be causing breast cancer.

By 2010, many doctors had been convinced by my arguments. In August 2010, a headline appeared in the *Independent* newspaper which shouted: ``Breast cancer screening harms as many women as it helps,' say doctors.' In late July 2011, a group of international cancer experts who had studied the effectiveness of breast cancer concluded that breast cancer screening programmes have `little detectable impact' on reducing death rates from the disease'. Today, it is widely accepted that mammography may be a major cause of breast cancer and is of very dubious value.

My fears about the danger of breast screening aren't my only concern with mammography.

Medical screening programmes can produce two types of error: false negatives and false positives. A false negative occurs when the screening programme misses a genuine cancer. For example, one in four breast cancers goes undetected by mammography. And a false positive occurs when the screening programme picks up what appears to be a cancer in a healthy breast.

Both types of error are acknowledged problems in all screening programmes. Breast screening programmes are certainly not exempt.

When there is a false negative result the main danger is obviously that a condition requiring treatment will be missed. But there is also a risk that the woman concerned may ignore - or dismiss - a lump which she feels in the bath, when dressing or when examining her own breasts because she has been given an official `all clear'.

False positives can lead to unnecessary tests, surgery, mutilation and potentially lethal chemotherapy.

A major Swedish survey (involving 600,000 women aged between 50 and 60) has shown that official breast screening did not produce any significant reduction in fatalities. Astonishingly, the Swedish survey showed that 100,000 of the 600,000 Swedish women had been falsely diagnosed as having cancer. Of these 16,000 had undergone biopsy and more than 400 had surgery - including mastectomy. In addition, of course, all those 100,000 women (and their partners) will have been exposed to tremendous anxiety and stress - and many immune systems will have been damaged as a result (ironically, increasing the likelihood of cancer developing).

In the UK, the medical establishment's response to this astonishing new evidence was not to call for official breast screening programmes to be stopped, or even to be reassessed, but to call for the breast screening programmes to be extended to include more women - and more screening. (This is the usual response when the truth tends to threaten a profitable medical enterprise.)

Many doctors believe that although sophisticated screening systems are now available for testing women's breasts the best way a woman can protect herself is to feel her own breasts regularly - preferably once a week or once a month. Indeed, figures show that despite huge expenditure on screening equipment 90% of breast cancer is discovered by women themselves.

Why, when the evidence shows so clearly that medical screening is a waste of time, does the medical establishment remain so enthusiastic?

Every independent survey I have found has concluded that screening (whether general or specific) is costly and useless. The reality is that the only people who benefit from screening programmes are doctors - and other parts of the health industry. Screening programmes are extremely profitable.

I find it difficult to avoid the conclusion that the medical profession (and the wider medical industry) remain enthusiastic about screening - despite the evidence - simply because medical screening is a hugely profitable business. Screening campaigns are often promoted by companies (and doctors) who make money out of them and if a company or clinic promotes medical screening you can be pretty sure that they aren't going to tell you the downside, or explain that it might, just might, do more harm than good.

For example, prostate cancer awareness week campaigns are sometimes promoted by companies making screening tests. These tests are expensive and they produce a mass of false positives and false negatives. The men with false positives think they have prostate cancer when they haven't. They worry a great deal. Worse still, they are treated by doctors and surgeons who also erroneously think they have prostate cancer. The men with false negatives walk away thinking they're perfectly healthy and can happily ignore any physical signs which they might develop.

The problems, and hazards, with screening programmes seem boundless. For example, you have a one in three chance of a false positive result if you have a full body CT scan. There is also a one in 20 chance that the scan will miss signs of disease - and give you a false sense of complacency and encourage you to ignore important physical signs.

In 2005, Brian Bulroney, the former Canadian Prime Minister went to the doctor for a routine check up. The check up included a CT scan which showed two small nodules. The former Prime Minister had surgery to have the nodules removed. Post-operatively he developed pancreatitis. He spent a month and a half in hospital and was discharged to recover at home. A month later he had to be readmitted because of a complication involving his pancreatitis.

Another month in hospital. There was nothing wrong with the nodules, by the way. They were harmless.

I've been screaming about the dangers of screening programmes for 30 years or more and was delighted when, in November 2009 the American Cancer Society finally accepted that screening for breast and prostate cancer is inefficient, inaccurate and alarmist and can do damage by detecting cancers that either don't exist or wouldn't kill if they did. Naturally, however, such programmes are still promoted within the NHS where staff favour screening programmes because it is easy to measure the results. They can say: `We screened 10,000 people and found 10 people with possible cancer. We, have, therefore, saved 10 lives.' In medical and statistical terms such claims are nonsensical. But in political terms they are invaluable.

The truth is that within the NHS the staff prefer organised screening programmes to proper preventive medicine because they are easier to organise and measure and because it is easy for the NHS to claim some credit for saving lives. Simply offering sensible advice is much cheaper and safer but the results cannot be measured and it is difficult for the NHS to claim the credit for saving lives.

Finally, here's my personal experience of routine screening.

Back in the 1980s I had to have an insurance medical. It was the usual, routine sort of thing but when performing a standard, simple screening test on my urine the doctor performing the medical found a trace of blood. I'd also been getting pains in my back and so the doctor referred me to the local hospital for investigations.

The hospital took X-rays and ultrasound pictures and two radiologists came to the conclusion that I had cancer of the kidney. If you're going to choose a cancer this isn't one that would be near the top of the list. It tends to be pretty lethal. The radiologists wanted to refer me to a surgeon straight away but I wanted a third opinion. I didn't feel happy with the diagnosis (and not just for the obvious reason) and somehow I just didn't feel that I needed to have a kidney ripped out.

After a scan it became clear that I didn't have cancer of the kidney. I had a slightly deformed kidney but there was nothing wrong with it. The two radiologists had been wrong.

So, what had caused the haematuria (blood in my urine)?

I made the diagnosis myself on a flight to Paris. As the air pressure in the cabin changed I started to suffer from the pain I'd been getting in my back. And I realised that the pain was caused by air in my intestine. I had irritable bowel syndrome caused largely by stress. The air in my bowel had been pressing on my kidneys and had caused the minute amount of bleeding.

I managed to get the irritable bowel syndrome under control and when I went back to the doctor for a second urine test he found that the haematuria had gone.

That was my first (and only) unhappy experience with a screening test. (I sent a letter detailing my observation to the *British Medical Journal* but they didn't print it. A decade later IBS was eventually recognised as a possible cause of haematuria.)

Last month I received an invitation to have a routine test for bowel cancer. The NHS wanted me to send in a stool sample which would be tested for blood as part of the NHS Bowel Cancer Screening Programme. If blood were found they would perform a colonoscopy.

I said 'no' because I was worried that the screening programme could kill me.

Here's the scenario that filled my mind.

The IBS (which still flares up) results in there being a little blood in my stools. The NHS screening test finds the blood and so I'm called in for a colonoscopy.

Now, one of the hazards with a colonoscopy is that the tube that is pushed up the bowel can puncture the bowel wall. It seemed to me that this is especially likely to happen if the wall is unusual, stretched or weakened. As it would undoubtedly be in someone with irritable bowel syndrome.

So the colonoscopy tube punctures my bowel wall.

Bang.

I need surgery. I need a hospital stay. I develop MRSA. And I die.

I decided that I would prefer to trust myself and that I would simply keep a look out for signs and symptoms of bowel cancer.

37. Will No One Rid Me Of The Lawyers?

I read the other day that a fat man was suing the NHS for allowing him to get fat. If he wins, the doors will be open and everyone with a health issue will consult a lawyer. Don't lawyers understand just how much they can damage the world with lawsuits like this? Actually, that's a stupid, rhetorical question because they obviously don't.

Nearly 40 years ago I wrote warning about the damage lawyers were doing to medical practice.

I was not concerned with patients receiving damages for injuries sustained as a result of genuine iatrogenic incidents but with lawyers representing patients who were creating claims out of thin air. I was also concerned about lawyers charging huge fees - all paid for out of money that should have been used to help patients.

It is right and proper that patients who have suffered genuine damage as a result of carelessness or error should be compensated.

But we have moved far, far beyond that state of affairs.

The big problem today is the existence of End Conditional Fee Agreements (popularly known as `no win, no fee' agreements).

Imported from America (together with other unpleasant inventions such as barbed wire and pantyhose, and quickly followed with a convenient change in the rules allowing lawyers to advertise for customers) these wretched legal devices account for half of the lawsuits against the NHS.

When these lawsuits are successful solicitors can claim up to 100% more than their original costs. It is wrong that solicitors should receive payments out of all proportion to the amount of damages awarded. In recent years, in those litigated no-win-no-fee cases where the average damages were Ł5,000 the average costs paid to the claimants' solicitors were Ł22,000. Even in claims resolved before proceedings were issued (where, logically, legal costs should be much lower) the average costs paid were almost double the damages paid. Lawyers are bleeding the NHS dry.

In one recent year the NHS paid out Ł248 million in compensation for medical 'blunders'. Plus another Ł134 million in costs.

Greedy lawyers are doing the same to commercial firms and all other public bodies. We could halt this trend in its tracks simply by making no-win-no-fee cases illegal. Allowing lawyers to work this way was an utter disaster in America and it has been an utter disaster in Britain, bringing endless misery to everyone except the lawyers.

The money lawyers take out of the health service is bad enough but it isn't the main problem. The real disaster is that today, as a result of the fear of litigation, doctors are increasingly unwilling to make diagnoses on the basis of clinical information. All the best doctors I knew when I was training made diagnoses after talking to and examining their patients. There was always a large element of intuition involved.

38. Medical Journalists: Bought And Paid For

The vast majority of medical journalists (whether medically qualified or not) report the views of the drug companies, academics (who are usually owned by drug companies) and medical establishment (ditto) quite uncritically and almost always without investigating the facts. It is for this reason that medical journalists hardly ever expose problematic drugs or procedures until the dangers are so blindingly obvious that the drugs or procedures have been withdrawn and replaced (usually by something equally poorly tested and equally unsafe). And it is for this reason that medical journalists never report the truth about vaccines, cancer, antibiotic therapy, radiotherapy, psychotherapy, animal experimentation or almost anything else you can think of.

Journalists who write about medicine get things wrong because they rely on doctors for their information. And, since doctors don't usually know the truth, journalists inevitably get misled too. Medical reporters usually believe what they are told by bureaucrats, drug company employees and grant-hungry academics. Most make no attempt to check or question what they are told because they don't know how to check or question the self-serving nonsense they are fed. Most medical journalists are unable to read scientific papers properly and incapable of asking the right questions. Even if they knew the questions to ask they wouldn't know what to do with the answers.

Bad products, bad doctors and bad companies are routinely praised. And in return the drug companies pay medical journalists obscenely large fees to write articles for their in-house magazines and to give presentations at rather snazzy luncheons and dinners. Sadly, newspapers (which tend to carry an enormous amount of job advertising for NHS staff and pharmaceutical advertising) are often reluctant to carry stories about NHS malpractice or medicinal drug related problems.

Medical journalists rarely seem to know anything very much about the subjects on which they profess to be experts. Almost every day I read reports in which journalists excitedly describe `new' discoveries which aren't new at all. Most of the `new' discoveries are, in reality, at least 20 years old. The problem (as I explained in my second book *Paper Doctors* in 1976) is that scientists and researchers are now producing so much (allegedly) new information that it is almost impossible for anyone to tell which is new and which merely repeats research which was done decades earlier. Journalists, submerged under a barrage of press releases, rarely have the time or the inclination to study old books, journals and newspapers.

Even official bodies are constantly repeating existing work, and issuing warnings that should have been acted upon decades earlier. For example, the effectiveness of some over-the-counter cough and cold medicines for children under 12 was questioned on 28th February 2009 in a review by the Medicines and Healthcare Products Regulatory Agency which found `no robust evidence' that many popular remedies work in children. (I offered the same criticism in my book *The Home Pharmacy* in 1980). In January 2011, it was officially reported that traffic noise could lead to an increase in the incidence of stress. (I published the same warning in *Stress Control* in 1978). Official review bodies are constantly warning that the NHS wastes money on buying branded drugs (I first made this point in

The Medicine Men in 1975). In one recent week I read that the incidence of tuberculosis was increasing rapidly (largely because drugs are prescribed in strengths not recommended by international guidelines), that children should be allowed to have *some* contact with germs because it would build up their immune system, that an obsession with cleanliness is a reason for the increase in allergies and infections, that food additives can be dangerous and that skin cancer among young women is on the rise and believed to be linked to the use of sun beds. I had published all these warnings in the 1970s - between 30 and 40 years earlier.

It seems that neither doctors nor journalists bother to read much history. I full expect to open one of the national broadsheets any day soon and discover that someone has invented a round device which they intend to call the 'wheel'.

In my second book *Paper Doctors* I noted that we would be much better off if, instead of paying for researchers to make 'new' discoveries and constantly searching for 'new' drugs we spent a little more time taking practical advantage of the information we have already acquired.

Sadly, it is difficult to create 'news' out of such a philosophy.

39. Big Brother's Evil Plan: Britain's NHS Computer Database

Everything the NHS does is expensive and incompetently managed. If NHS employees do one thing well it is `waste money'. For some years now the NHS has been quietly planning a huge database designed to contain private medical information about every citizen in the country. (Though, naturally, I suspect that the private medical information relating to important politicians and their relatives will be excluded on `security' grounds.)

Upgrading the NHS computer system has been described as the biggest civilian computer project in the world. It has also been described as the world's biggest civil IT failure. The whole absurd and pointless white elephant has cost so many billions that no one seems quite certain how much has been spent. It is utterly improper, unethical and unnecessary and back in 2006 I described it as doomed to inglorious failure.

The bureaucrats have always claimed, of course, that our personal medical information will be well-protected from snoopers.

There will, say expensively paid bureaucrats, be firewalls to stop hackers finding out how many times you've been depressed or infected with an embarrassing disease.

Ha ha.

Do the bureaucrats really believe that they can create firewalls which will keep hackers out?

Hackers have even got into the Pentagon's top secret computers. There is no computer system in the world which cannot be hacked into. Announcing that a system is super-safe merely provides hackers with a super-challenge.

But that's not the real problem.

The real problem is that when your private medical records (the things you told your doctor in confidence) are put onto the computer, nothing about you will really be private again.

When I first declared the project doomed (five years before the authorities admitted that the scheme was stuffed), the NHS had already registered 298,973 staff members as being entitled to have access to our confidential medical records. But that, of course, was just the beginning. There will be more. Millions more. Pharmacists (and the assistants working in the chemist's shop) will have access to our information. Hundreds of thousands of clerks and administrators in the NHS will have access to our personal medical history. Every secret we have shared with our doctors will be there for everyone to read.

The information will, naturally, be made available to drug companies. (They say they need the personal information for testing drugs. Phooey. They want it for drug marketing. Once the drug companies get hold of our information they will, for example, have the name, age and home address of every diabetic patient in the country. And the names and addresses of all other patients with specific disorders. Pure marketing gold.)

Social workers, policemen and local authority workers will also all demand access to the computer. And they will get it. Once every policeman in the country can read about our depressions, our irritable bowel syndromes and our miscarriages then our last vestige of privacy will be lost. For ever. Everyone you meet or know who works for the Government (and everyone you meet or know who knows someone who works for the Government) will know everything that is in our medical records. Everything we've ever told our doctors. Everything we ever tell them in the future. The Government should have saved its money and just put the nation's medical records onto Facebook. It would have been just as confidential, and infinitely cheaper.

Today, I often complain that many doctors don't take confidentiality seriously. But does anyone seriously expect policemen and social workers to regard confidentiality as important?

GPs, not usually too worried about the rights of patients, have already expressed disquiet. A poll has shown that a majority of family doctors fear that the system will be vulnerable to hackers and to public officials who don't need access to confidential information. They worry that what is left of the doctor-patient relationship will disappear and that more and more people will refuse to discuss delicate issues with their doctor.

(I believe that confidentiality is vital. Over a quarter of a century ago I resigned as a GP when NHS bureaucrats tried to force me to write confidential information about my patients on sick notes. I refused and was fined heavily for doing so. It seemed to me that this was a vital matter of principle. Patients are entitled to believe that what they tell their doctors in confidence will remain confidential. I felt that by putting diagnoses on sick notes (likely to be read by heaven knows how many people) I would be betraying that confidence. And so I resigned from the NHS and became a full-time writer.)

Patients who want to stop all this happening, and who don't want to have their personal medical history put onto the Government's computer, are to be told that they must write to their GP. And GPs have been told that they must forward all letters from patients who want to opt out of the central NHS computer system. The letters must be sent on the Secretary of State. Yes, your private letter to your GP must be forwarded (with or without your consent) to the Government.

So that they know who you are. And where you live.

Presumably, so that they can give you a black mark.

Back in 2006, before such economic luminaries as Gordon Brown and Fred Goodwin took us on a long and painful journey into national bankruptcy, `they' reckoned the official bill for the NHS computer had risen to Ł20 billion. (That was the official figure so it was probably double that.) That was Ł333 for every man, woman and child in Britain. Billions spent on a computer system which we don't want and which probably won't ever work and which will destroy what remains of our privacy. But by mid May 2011, when even the politicians and the bureaucrats had decided that the system was a failure, it was announced that the Government had spent just

Ł2.7 billion on the project. (They presumably hoped that no one had kept a record of the previous estimate.) It was then officially announced that the system was not cost effective and wasn't going to work.

The new system has already caused 110 major computer incidents in hospitals in just four months. Lives have been put at risk after essential hospital computer systems crashed as a result of this project. And, of course, there have been errors. For example, one patient was wrongly listed on the computer as being an alcoholic.

Wouldn't all that money be better spent on getting rid of long waiting lists, dirty wards, single sex wards and so on?

Doctors don't want this super register of patients' illnesses. There is no logical medical need for it. It will mean an end to patient confidentiality.

It was always obvious that the scheme would create problems rather than solve them. But there was, of course, a hidden agenda. The plan was to put our medical records onto the new NHS computer so that the Government could feed all the information onto our new Identity Cards. When the ID card system fell apart the need for the national NHS data system also fell apart.

The inescapable truth is that every large organisation which has computerised its records has made life unbearably difficult for customers and staff. I give you British Gas, British Telecom, Britain's entire rail system and HMRC as examples of chaos caused by computerisation designed to make life simpler. It isn't the computers which cause the problem, of course. It's the millions of lazy, incompetent, half-witted zombies who design the software, input the information and then struggle to retrieve it. The evidence to date suggests that any computerised NHS records system will be, from every conceivable point of view, an unmitigated disaster. But then, that shouldn't be too much of a surprise to anyone who has watched the bizarre growth of the new `information technology' industry. The bald truth is that the communications industry has benefited only the communications industry. Everything worked better, more efficiently and more economically before computers.

If we must use computers, then the obvious way to use a national computer to our advantage is to use it to record drug side effects. I've been advocating this since the seventies. It would be simple to organise. Doctors would merely key in details of side effects they'd noticed, or that patients had reported. Even patients could be encouraged to add information. And so, within days of new drugs being introduced, potentially dangerous side effects would be clear. Doctors could be warned. Deadly drugs could be withdrawn. Thousands of lives would be saved.

I first advocated this simple, relatively inexpensive use of the computer four decades ago. But finding side effects at an early stage would not be in the interests of the drug companies. And so it would not suit the unholy trinity. And so it won't happen.

40. Complaints Not Wanted

The number of complaints made about the NHS is rising constantly and repeatedly breaking new records. In a strange way, however, I confess that I am delighted. Only if people complain about the service they receive will politicians and doctors sit up and take notice.

At the moment however, the problem is that the complaints procedure doesn't work - and is, indeed, designed to protect staff members rather than patients and is, for all practical purposes, entirely pointless. For example, the NHS is obsessed with protecting staff from injury. Time and time again I have heard about hospitals where nurses refuse to lift or move patients in case they hurt their backs. Well, I'm afraid that is what the job entails and nurses who can't be bothered to learn how to lift properly should do something else for a living. Hospitals which concentrate on issues like this, and ignore the problem of hospital infections, are mixing up their priorities. It all reminds me of the BP oil company which worried a good deal about making sure that people didn't go up and down stairs carrying cups of coffee but ran a sloppy system which led to major disasters.

In 2010, more than 100,000 people made written complaints about NHS hospitals and community services. Patients (and their relatives) complained about both the treatment that had been provided and the attitude of staff. Years of targets and box ticking have done nothing to improve the NHS but have merely protected the staff against censure.

Red tape, political correctness, litigation and a mass of bizarre rules and regulations have wrecked the way hospitals operate. Hospital staff who make egregious errors cannot be punished - let alone told off - because of new employment rules which are weighted dispiritingly in favour of the employee. New EU laws mean that the hours junior doctors spend sleeping must now be counted as time worked. The result is that there are nowhere near enough doctors to go around. And so nurses are being allowed to prescribe drugs and perform minor surgery. In my view nurses aren't trained or equipped to prescribe drugs. Doctors, who are supposed to trained, make enough mistakes.

The complaints that are made produce no improvement for several reasons. When criticisms about the NHS are aired there is invariably a flood of protest from 'satisfied' patients and relatives who are, presumably, too stupid to know what they should expect a hospital to be like, or who have been coerced into writing by relatives who work for the NHS. No one who knows what a hospital should do could possibly be satisfied with the NHS. Nevertheless, every attempt to make real changes has so far been thwarted by undemanding people whose expectations are set somewhere in the darkest part of the Middle Ages. Patients and families who stick up for and defend the NHS on the basis of an isolated personal experience help to perpetuate the problems. Intelligent, caring people should always support those criticising an institution or the people working in the institution become complacent. Patients and relatives think and say that they are pleased or satisfied because they don't know what to expect, or how to judge the quality of the treatment they receive. The only people who think the NHS is wonderful are the ones who have become accustomed to awful care and regard it as acceptable. Clever propaganda convinces victims that they are beneficiaries. I'm afraid that NHS patients who write complimentary letters about the NHS to their local paper are doing more harm than good. They are encouraging the survival of a stagnant, rancid system which kills patients and destroys the souls, spirits and integrity of doctors and nurses. It's like someone who was in Auschwitz whooping about the excellent conditions because they were befriended by a guard and given an extra biscuit. Everyone who says that the NHS is wonderful is killing someone else.

NHS staff have learned that if they follow the letter of the law, and obey all the administrative regulations, it doesn't matter a damn how they treat the patients. Staff are only ever fired if they are convicted of the mass murder of patients. Well over a million people work for the NHS and they have a vested interest in it remaining inefficient. They work too little and are paid too much. Targets are designed so that the system can announce its own successes, but the needs of patients are ignored and their cries of dissatisfaction are stifled. There are too many administrators and the whole health service is suffocating under red tape. The NHS isn't going to get any better because its primary aim now is to look after its staff rather than to look after the people who use it. The whole institution (like all State run-institutions) has been manipulated and adapted so that the requirements and rights and interests of the staff are put first. Commercial organisations (such as private hospitals) cannot survive if they operate in this way, but State-run organisations can do so very well because the link between the person paying the bills, and the people being paid for providing the service, has been broken.

It has become standard practice for hospitals to take a long time in dealing with complaints. They have learnt a lot from insurance companies. Their philosophy is that if you let things meander along then eventually most of the people complaining will die, go away, get bored or just become too exhausted to carry on. If you make a complaint about an NHS employee, the bureaucrats move smoothly into action. At the very best you will get letters thanking you for your concern and assuring you that they are constantly reviewing their procedures. No one dares apologise because they're worried about being sued. And so the same mistakes are made time and time again. (Doctors and nurses are so terrified of being sued that much medical practice is now governed not by what is right medically, or what makes common sense, but by the potential requirements of lawyers in the courtroom.)

Within the modern NHS no one takes any blame for things that go wrong. Everyone has an excuse, a reason, for the error they've made. And when there is no obvious excuse there is always the computer. NHS staff have learned from politicians and sportsmen: when something goes wrong it isn't their fault. Staff everywhere are being taught to take no responsibility. (How can you do anything wrong, if you weren't responsible for what you did?) And, of course, large organisations always exist for meetings and National Health Service meetings, organised by bureaucrats, nurses and social workers, exist to provide a sense of importance and a reason for their own existence. The short-term aim is not to make decisions but, rather, to *avoid* making any decisions. The long-term aim is to ensure that another meeting can be arranged, the sense of self-importance sustained and the responsibility for making the wrong decision avoided.

The NHS is run for staff rather than patients and the sole aim is to satisfy bureaucratic targets and to provide secure, undemanding employment for large numbers of people. The NHS exists to provide secure employment for a vast army of jobsworths. Gordon Brown, whose target culture destroyed Britain's public services, has, I believe, destroyed what was left of the NHS, and the NHS won't improve until it is in the interests of the staff to change things.

Moreover, with standards so low in the NHS, private care will continue to deteriorate.

Another problem is that medical records have a tendency to disappear whenever a patient makes a complaint. And without records it is very difficult to pursue a complaint to any sensible conclusion. Where do the medical records go to? `Do hospitals have a special person who gets rid of them?' asked my wife, Donna Antoinette. And I couldn't help wondering if they do. Perhaps all Government establishments now have a Senior Administrative Officer (Shredding) whose job it is to get rid of anything which might prove embarrassing or expensive. After my father died his hospital medical records were missing for ages. They eventually turned up in a cupboard in a nursing home.

NHS complaints should be investigated by independent experts. There are thousands of retired doctors and nurses who could do this job brilliantly well.

And maybe what all health systems need is some sort of points system - such as the one used by the police for speeding motorists. Staff members who make mistakes could be given points. If they collect too many points they could be fined and suspended. Or executed. (That's what they would probably do in China.)

Incidentally, the people who worry that they will be left unprotected if the NHS disappears should realise that if the NHS were closed, and the money which we now spend on it used to buy private care health insurance for the whole population, there would be billions of pounds left over with which to buy sickness insurance for every man, woman and child so that everyone would be insured against financial loss when needing to take time off work through illness. That's how bad and wasteful the NHS is today.

41. The General Medical Council Is Worse Than Useless

When doctors are believed to have erred, the ultimate complaints procedure involves the General Medical Council (GMC), an organisation which regulates doctors and is supposed to protect patients from bad doctors. The GMC decides whether or not doctors are fit to practise. And it lays down rules and guidelines detailing how they should practise and how they should treat their patients.

But if the GMC really exists to protect the health of patients, and the integrity and reputation of the medical profession (and, if it does not, then why does it exist?), then in my view it has failed both doctors and patients.

Here are ten ways in which I believe that the GMC has failed patients and doctors:

1. The GMC does nothing to limit the enormous control the drug companies have over medical education. The GMC has stood by while the medical profession has been taken over by an industry. As I wrote in *The Medicine Men* in 1976, `a profession which takes its instructions from an industry can no longer call itself a profession'. A GMC which truly cared about professional standards would punish doctors who, while practising medicine, develop over-close links with drug companies. Doctors and drug companies have (or should have) completely different aims.

2. The GMC allows doctors to overprescribe drugs such as antibiotics and tranquillisers without publishing adequate guidelines and without punishing the thousands of doctors who recklessly

overprescribe. The overprescribing of tranquillisers has led to the biggest addiction problem in Britain. The overprescribing of antibiotics has contributed to the incidence of antibiotic-resistant infections in hospitals.

3. The GMC does nothing to ensure that doctors only provide patients with the best possible advice. After a GP was reported to have `prescribed' meat for his patients, I made a formal complaint about him to the GMC on the grounds that meat is a recognised cause of cancer. (The scientific evidence for this is published on www.vernoncoleman.com). Despite the existence of this evidence the GMC refused to take any action against the GP.

4. The GMC has made no criticism of the way the NHS (the main source of health care in Britain) is mismanaged by politicians and administrators. There is little or no point in the GMC admonishing doctors for breaches of medical etiquette when the environment in which they work is dangerously and criminally inadequate. It is simply not good enough for the GMC to say that the medical environment in which doctors operate is not its concern. That is akin to a GP treating patients poisoned by a pollutant and doing nothing to eradicate the pollutant on the grounds that it isn't his responsibility. If the GMC is to be taken seriously it must tackle serious issues.

5. The GMC has done nothing to prevent doctors taking advantage of the existence of two different health systems (the NHS and private care) in order to make money. Thousands of British doctors work both for the NHS and for their own interests. Many of them deliberately make their NHS waiting lists long so that they can attract more private patients. It is improper and unethical for doctors who work for the NHS to offer private care to the same pool of patients. The GMC should interfere and stop this abuse.

6. The GMC should do more to prevent the abuse of minority groups of patients, such as those who are mentally ill and those who are elderly. Doctors who withhold treatment and allow patients to die just because they are old (a common practice in NHS hospitals) are not punished by the GMC. They should be. By refusing to

acknowledge the existence of this problem, and by refusing to do anything about it, the GMC is ignoring the needs of patients and abandoning its own fundamental responsibility.

7. The GMC should punish doctors who work in hospitals which have higher than average levels of antibiotic-resistant infection. Many British hospitals are dirty. This is why antibiotic-resistant infections are higher in Britain than almost anywhere else in the world. Neither administrators nor nurses will take responsibility for this tragic state of affairs and so doctors must. The GMC should question and monitor doctors whose hospitals are dirty, or which have a high incidence of MRSA infection, and should punish those doctors who do not insist that the appropriate changes are made in cleaning and nursing practices. It seems to me that the GMC doesn't much care if doctors kill their patients wholesale as long as they don't sleep with them retail.

8. The GMC should make it clear that medical confidentiality is of primary importance to the integrity of the doctor-patient relationship. Any doctor who is guilty of a breach of medical confidentiality should be struck off the medical register. You can't be a little bit confidential any more than you can be a little bit pregnant. Doctors should be instructed not to share confidential information with social workers, policemen, politicians, bureaucrats or anyone else who isn't directly concerned with the health of the patient concerned. Politicians and judges who attempt to overrule the principle of medical confidentiality should be advised that the GMC will not accept interference in this area. However, instead of promoting the importance of confidentiality the GMC seems to have fallen over backwards to ensure that confidentiality becomes a thing of the past. In September 2009, the GMC told doctors that they should share a range of confidential information with the `authorities'. Alarmed by this I sent the following letter to the GMC:

`I was surprised to hear that you have decided that in future I should break my Hippocratic Oath and tell the police if I treat a victim of a gun or knife crime. I was equally startled by your assertion that I can tell relatives about diagnoses of genetic disease and should tell social services if patients harm themselves. These are appalling

decisions which seem designed to destroy the very principle of confidentiality. Confidentiality is like pregnancy: it doesn't come in degrees. The doctor's primary responsibility must be to the patient he is treating and not to the public. When I qualified as a doctor I took the Hippocratic Oath. Who gave the GMC the right to decide that I should now break that solemn Oath?

These are appalling decisions (which seem to me to be politically motivated and contrary to Article 9 of the Human Rights Act) and no thinking doctor should obey them.

Although I am fully registered (and intend to remain registered and licensed) I will not obey your instruction to disobey the Hippocratic Oath and, indeed, I do not believe you have the moral right to demand that I do so.'

Over a month later I received a reply from someone called Jane O'Brien, (described as Assistant Director, Standards and Fitness to Practise Directorate). She told me: `We agree that doctors' first concern should be the patients they treat, and that a relationship of confidentiality is a key part of forming a relationship of trust in which the patient can receive good care. However, we do not see the duty of confidentiality (as) an absolute'.

So, the GMC believes it is possible to be a little bit pregnant. The bureaucrats at the GMC clearly don't realise that nothing a doctor tells the Government (or a State employee such as a policeman, tax inspector, local council employee, doctor, nurse or social worker) will be treated as confidential. The Government will either sell the information or lose it.

9. The GMC should look carefully at some of the more bizarre medical fashions. For example, it is surely wrong that surgeons should remove the breasts of healthy women, or should perform operations on patients suffering from nothing more than obesity caused by overeating. And the Government's enthusiasm for vaccination is not supported by convincing scientific evidence. Currently fashionable vaccination programmes may do more harm

than good. Doctors who advocate or promote vaccination programmes should be investigated by the GMC.

10. The GMC should make a clear statement about how medical research should be conducted. For example, the evidence clearly proves that reliance on animal experiments is one of the factors responsible for the current endemic of drug-induced disease. One in six patients in hospital is there because he or she has been made ill by a doctor. This is unacceptable. The Department of Health has been quite unable to produce any evidence supporting the use of animal experiments in medical research. The GMC should make it clear that drugs should be properly tested before being made available for general prescribing and that animal testing has no place in the development process for new drugs. Doctors who support or advocate animal testing should be investigated by the GMC.

11. The GMC should have spoken up when the Government accepted EU laws about doctors' working hours. The General Medical Council, which is supposed to spend its huge income preserving medical standards, should have realised the effect that reduced working weeks would have on patient care. However, the GMC, which was once a rather lumbering but reasonably reliable organisation run by the medical profession to maintain a register of all doctors and to dish out punishments to the bad ones, has become a political toy. It is, it seems to me, of no practical value to patients or doctors but of enormous practical value to politicians and bureaucrats. The GMC's main role today seems to be to create ever more complex rules and regulations to keep its bureaucrats busy and to justify its vast overheads. (Like many quangos and quango-like organisations the GMC also likes raising money, which it needs to pay the vast salaries of all the administrators it has acquired to help it raise more money. There are licence fees and registration fees and there will soon be revalidation fees and fees for doctors who want to go to the lavatory.) The GMC staff must realise that the EU's rules have devastated the quality of medical care in Britain. It could have insisted that the Government reject the absurd EU legislation. But, as far as I know, not an eyebrow or a voice was raised in protest. The bottom line is that the GMC is a multi-million pound money-making machine with plush offices in central London. And that's about it. I

believe it is self-serving and far too pro-establishment and that for all the good it does for patients and doctors it could be replaced by a single clerk equipped with a computer and a website. The GMC is a rich and hugely successful licensing body which seems to me to exist to collect money rather than to protect patients or defend the interests of doctors or to improve medical standards. It seems out of touch with reality and completely fails to understand the extent of the iatrogenesis problem.

The GMC will pillory and strike off a doctor found guilty of kissing, groping or propositioning a willing patient. But killing patients is fine, especially if they're old. The GMC launches investigations and then makes judgements. These are chiselled in stone. It is absurd to have a single body launching an investigation and then making a judgement. Patients and doctors deserve (and need) much more than an organisation which, like so many quangos, now seems to exist only to exist; a support agency for the unholy trinity of State, drug industry and medical establishment.

Today, the General Medical Council gives a false sense of security and leadership: it is far worse than useless. I believe that without it, many of the problems I have outlined would be tackled and put right.

42. How Lobbyists Buy Lives

One of the problems with the NHS is that the people who use it don't understand that the amount of money available for health care is finite. Lobby groups push for money for their small area and, inevitably, the lobby groups which are best organised get most of the money. Lobbyists and pressure groups exist to ensure that the available money is spent unfairly and unequally.

Powerful organisations campaigning for particular groups of patients put pressure on the controlling political party, and force the Government to provide treatment for their group. But this is done at the expense of other patients. And so fashionable, politically correct groups (such as those requiring infertility treatment) are treated, while the elderly (not at all fashionable or politically correct) are allowed to go blind and to die when they could be treated quite cheaply.

Breast cancer, which is fashionable and media friendly, receives enormous amounts of money. But less attractive areas (preventive medicine and bowel cancer for example) receive very little attention or funding. People use the Human Rights Act to help them get whatever they want out of the NHS. Foreigners come in and use the NHS freely; welcomed by administrators who do not seem to understand that even the vast amount of money the NHS receives is finite and that when money is spent on providing free breast enlargement surgery for Argentinians, some poor Britons with rectal bleeding will wait six months to see a specialist and may die because they weren't seen sooner. Every time someone has infertility treatment, or cosmetic surgery, someone somewhere dies of undiagnosed, untreated bowel cancer.

The lunacy which is the NHS seems unending. This morning I noticed in the news that a 39-year-old unemployed, single woman had Ł4,000 worth of IVF funded by the NHS. She wanted a baby and, not having a husband or even a boyfriend, considered that the NHS had to provide her with one. That's Ł4,000 not available to spend on saving someone with bowel cancer. And, the same day, there was news that a Nigerian woman who had taken infertility drugs, had come to the UK to have her quintuplets on the NHS. Why wouldn't you? Having quins would cost a fortune in Nigeria, America, France or Lithuania. The cost to the NHS? An estimated Ł200,000 and counting. How many taxpaying Britons will die because of *that*?

Everywhere you look it is clear that as a result of pressure from people promoting specific interests, NHS staff have helped create unfairness and favouritism. Britain is, for example, now a nation pandering to regiments of whingeing drug addicts. As anyone in the drug addiction business will confirm, cocaine and heroin are relatively non-addictive. It is much, much harder to kick tobacco, alcohol or, worst of all, benzodiazepine tranquillisers, than it is to get off cocaine or heroin. But people who got hooked on tranquillisers through no fault of their own receive little or no public help whereas people who acquired an illegal drug habit are spoilt with advisors, helpers and more money than they know what to do with.

And only the NHS could create an AIDS industry so large that it had more staff than patients. AIDS `experts' (who knew little or nothing about the disease) fought over patients, potential patients or possible patients. Why? Because there weren't enough patients around to justify all their various salaries.

43. When Simple Solutions Are Ignored

The NHS treats prostate cancer with drugs, radiotherapy or surgery. But one doctor (Dean Ornish) in America has shown that prostate cancer be treated with a simple regime which consists of moderate exercise, a vegan diet and stress relaxation techniques. Writing in the *Journal of Urology* Dr Ornish showed that patients who followed this regime rigorously saw their prostate antigen scores drop. Blood serum taken from patients on this programme inhibited cancer cells eight times as much as serum from other patients. And there seems no doubt that green vegetables and lycopene provide protection against cancer-promoting chemicals. But, despite this evidence, the NHS continues to treat prostate cancer with drugs, radiotherapy or surgery.

As I reported in *How To Stop Your Doctor Killing You* it is possible to treat serious heart disease without surgery by using a simple regime similar to this one. And it is also possible to treat diabetes with a similar programme.

Sadly, however, the NHS is now controlled by the pharmaceutical industry and consequently such safe, effective, patient-empowering and economical regimes are not favoured. It is hardly surprising that the NHS, once the dream of so many, once the justifiable envy of the world, has become a creaking hulk; misguided by navigators blinded by avarice, badly managed by an incompetent, lazy, greedy crew and allowed to founder on the twin rocks of ignorance and self-interest.

44. How The European Union Kills People

There is no doubt that one of the reasons why our health care system is a failure is because it is distorted by regulations, targets and legislation - some of which originate in London but much of which now comes from the European Union.

There is no doubt at all that the European Union has done enormous damage to the quality of medical care provided to patients in Europe. It is, for example, because of the EU that general practitioners in England no longer provide 24 hour cover for their patients and it is because of the EU that hospital patients rarely see the same doctor twice and may often go for several days (particularly over weekends and bank holidays) without seeing a doctor at all.

It was back in the 1990s that European politicians and bureaucrats insisted that the European working-time directive should be applied to doctors as well as to coach drivers and factory workers. This was done purely for political reasons.

Britain accepted the EU rules for doctors. (The Government could have refused to accept the legislation but it didn't. As our politicians always do, our ministers bowed to the EU's demands.) One reason for the acceptance of the new legislation was, without doubt, the fact that there will, as a result of sexual discrimination, soon be far more women than men in medicine. Women doctors are far less likely to be driven by vocation and altruistic motives and far more likely to want as much money as possible for as little work as possible. Women doctors marry, have babies and want to work office hours. Just like female MPs, they demanded a regulated 'work-life balance' and expected the job commitments to be adjusted to suit them. They aren't prepared to give the commitment that male doctors have always given. And so patients lack continuity and male doctors have to work harder. The result has been the worst and fastest deterioration in the NHS since its inception in 1948.

Today, the entire NHS is in a mess. Doctors no longer provide patients with anything like half-way decent medical care, and patients die like wasps in autumn because the quality of care has deteriorated. There is no longer any continuity of care.

Thanks largely to the EU employment rules, doctors in hospital (as in general practice) are now working strictly limited hours. Many GPs no longer provide the 24 hour, 365 day service which was an integral part of family practice just a few years ago. The modern GP works the sort of hours usually associated with school teachers, librarians and accountants. Similarly, many hospital doctors now work only short, fixed weeks. Hospital doctors who are 'on call' are deemed to be working when they are sleeping.

At the same time, the EU has taken rights away from patients and given lots of new rights to employees. The result is that staff everywhere have all the power and can be as rude as they like without censure.

Today, if hospital doctors work more hours than the EU permits then the hospital must pay a huge fine. (In exactly the same way that the EU controls the amount and type of rubbish our councils can collect so doctors working hours are now controlled precisely by the EU.) The result of this bureaucratic absurdity is that doctors have to leave half way through treating patients and at weekends hospitals are often completely empty of doctors. I wonder how many patients have died as a result of this policy? I'm damned sure it is considerably more than ever died as a result of doctors being tired. Today it is rare to see a doctor (or a physiotherapist or, indeed, anyone else who isn't a patient or a visitor) in a hospital at weekends. Patients are left lying in bed for over two days. No one, it seems, has heard of deep vein thromboses or pressure sores.

Today, hospitals don't discharge patients at the weekend because consultants aren't available. And they know that if they send patients home at the weekend they will have empty beds and will have to accept new patients - something they don't like doing over weekends with a skeleton medical staff in the hospital.

Another result of the shortage of doctors has been that nurses have been given the right to prescribe and to perform surgery - and to take on these responsibilities without proper medical supervision and without the sort of training required for doctors. To the problem of bad prescribing by doctors has now been added the problem of bad prescribing by nurses. Most nurses (like most doctors) know very little about the drugs they prescribe and know next to nothing about side effects. We need fewer - not more - people handing out prescriptions.

To make sure that doctors stick to the EU's regulations hospitals now employ highly-paid bureaucrats whose sole job is to make sure that young doctors clock off on time and don't spend a moment more than they should looking after patients. Hospitals employ Working Time Directive Project Managers (salaries around Ł40,000 a year) whose job description involves 'ensuring the compliance of young professionals with the 48 hour working limit'.

So, with one thing and another, it is hardly surprising that it is often difficult to find a doctor on a hospital ward these days. And it is hardly surprising that the standard of care in our hospitals has fallen and is still falling rapidly.

And it is hardly surprising that more and more patients are getting fed up with the poor quality of care they receive from doctors. In 2007, the number of complaints heard by the General Medical Council was 20 times as great as it had been in 1997. (Incidentally, a high proportion of the complaints relate to services provided by foreign born doctors. Naturally, no one is allowed to mention this although it has been the case for some years.)

Forcing the EU working directive into the world of medicine has created one other massive problem.

When doctors qualified in the 1970s, specialists only became consultants or GPs after around 30,000 hours of experience and training. In 1971, when I was a junior hospital doctor I worked all the hours available. It was not uncommon for a junior house officer to be on duty for 168 hours a week, snatching hours of sleep whenever there was a lull in activity. We didn't complain about this because it was an accepted part of our training and, being young, we managed perfectly well. Every patient was looked after by a designated consultant team. The consultant, registrar and house officer were responsible for patients from their admittance to their discharge. The extraordinary workload meant that young, resident doctors learned an enormous amount about practical, medical care. Today, thanks to reduced working hours, young doctors can become consultants or fully qualified GPs after 6,000 hours of training. So, today's specialists have one fifth the experience of their predecessors just 30 years ago. How can that possibly be acceptable? If airline pilots were suddenly allowed to fly passenger planes after a training period that had been cut by four fifths there would be a public outcry.

45. Looking To The Future

There is no role for State-run medicine today. It has been proven to be neither cost-effective nor advantageous for patients. In Britain, the NHS should be allowed to die. It was always a terrible idea. Nothing the Government runs ever works. This is because politicians make useless managers, while the people they employ don't care enough about what they do to make any effort to do it half decently. The best (or worst) example of the failure of politicians and public employees to run anything effectively is the National Health Service.

The Government (encouraged by the fascist arch-enemy of all goodness, the European Union) spends vast amounts of our money creating illness and causing profitable epidemics. They encourage meat eating - now the biggest cause of cancer in the Western world. They prevent people from finding out the truths about the food they buy. They allow advertising that is as manipulative as it is dishonest. And then they throw up their hands in astonishment as the incidence of heart disease, cancer and obesity all rocket. Our present system actively encourages ill health.

In Britain the NHS needs reforming. But that's just one small part of the problem. What we really need is a reform of our entire approach to life and health. We need a physical revolution, a mental revolution and a spiritual revolution.

The NHS is a bureaucratic monster which kills more people than it saves. It is absurdly expensive, wasteful and inefficient. There are more administrators than nurses or beds. The annual cost of NHS management is an outrageous and indefensible Ł12.6 billion. That's double the amount the NHS spends on accident and emergency services, dental services and maternity care. To describe the NHS as an expensive and dangerous disaster is to understate the situation. If you are taken ill the chances are that it will not be the illness that will kill you but the treatment you receive afterwards. We would, as a nation, be better off with nothing. If that sounds overstated, it isn't.

Some people are saved, of course. Road accident victims and patients requiring emergency surgery may have reason to thank the NHS for their lives. But thousands more are damaged or killed by poor prescribing, inaccurate diagnoses, dangerous vaccines, incompetent nursing and so on. As a doctor who has studied the consequences of iatrogenesis I don't think it is any exaggeration to say that the NHS now kills more people than it saves.

Anyone who enters an NHS hospital as a patient is putting their life at risk. If cigarette packets deserve to carry a health warning then so do hospitals.

Replacing the NHS with a system of private medical care would employ far fewer bureaucrats but it would be infinitely fairer and better and considerably cheaper.

Don't believe me? Look at the figures.

We spend around Ł104 billion a year on the NHS.

There are around 60,000,000 people in the UK.

Divide 60,000,000 into Ł104 billion.

And you have around Ł1,750 per head.

I could buy damned good private health cover for Ł1,750 year. And so could you.

And yet no political party will ever dare suggest closing the NHS and replacing it with a private health care system. And so nothing in this book will change anything immediately.

But I've written this book and you've read it and so there are now at least two of us who know the truth. And that's a start.

Postscript 1: Coleman's Laws

Coleman's 1st Law Of Medicine

If you are receiving treatment for an existing disease and you develop new symptoms then, until proved otherwise, you should assume that the new symptoms are caused by the treatment you are receiving.

Coleman's 2nd Law Of Medicine

There is no point in having tests done unless the results will affect your treatment.

Coleman's 3rd Law Of Medicine

If the treatment doesn't work then you should consider the possibility that the diagnosis might be wrong. This is particularly true when several treatments have been tried.

Coleman's 4th Law Of Medicine

Screening examinations and check-ups are more profitable for doctors than for patients.

Coleman's 5th Law Of Medicine

It is doctors, not patients, who need annual check-ups.

Coleman's 6th Law Of Medicine

Hospitals are not suitable places for sick people. If you must go into one, you should get out as quickly as you can.

Coleman's 7th Law Of Medicine

There are fashions in medicine just as much as there are fashions in clothes. The difference is that whereas badly conceived fashions in clothes are only likely to embarrass you, ill-conceived fashions in medicine may kill you. The fashions in medicine have, by and large, as much scientific validity as the fashions in the rag trade.

Coleman's 8th Law Of Medicine

The medical establishment will always take decisions on health matters which benefit industry, Government and the medical profession, rather than patients. And the Government will always take decisions on health matters which benefit the State rather than individual patients. What you read or hear about medicine and health matters will have more to do with the requirements of the pharmaceutical industry and the Government, than the genuine needs of patients.

Coleman's 9th Law Of Medicine

Doctors and nurses know little or nothing about staying healthy. In particular, doctors and nurses know nothing useful about food, diet and healthy eating. (Sadly, the same is true of nutritionists and dieticians).

Coleman's 10th Law Of Medicine

There are no holistic healers. There are only holistic patients.

Coleman's 11th Law Of Medicine

There is no such thing as minor surgery.

Coleman's 12th Law Of Medicine

Some patients will always be treated more equally than others.

Taken from *Coleman's Laws* by Vernon Coleman

Postscript 2: An Interview with Vernon Coleman

Question 1.

You have been publishing books for over 30 years, initially books on medicine. Why and how did you get into publishing and did you initially expect to have sold over two million books?

Answer

I started writing books in the mid 1970s but I didn't start publishing them myself until the late 1980s. I'd written a book which purported to be a diary of a cat - called *Alice's Diary*. My literary agent at the time tried all my usual publishers in London. None of them would consider it. `Who would buy a book by a cat?' said some disdainfully. `Vernon doesn't write cat books,' sniffed others. So I published it myself. Every year since then the book has sold enough copies to have been constantly on and off the hardback bestseller lists for fiction. (It hasn't, of course, actually been on the bestseller lists. The publishing industry doesn't work like that.) After that I published a few more books. And then I started buying back the rights to books which had been published by other publishers. So, for example, I bought back the rights to a book of mine called *Bodypower* which had gone straight into the *Sunday Times* Top Ten when it first came out in the early 1980s - published by a smart London publisher. But modern publishers don't bother much with back list titles and so ten years later it wasn't doing much. The paperback publisher was selling hardly any copies. I bought up their stock (which had a dull looking cover) and gave them away so that I could get the rights back. *Bodypower* has been selling in thousands ever since. Now I publish my books in the UK and sell the rights to foreign publishers, to audio publishers and so on.

Question 2.

Were your early books successful?

Answer

The first book I ever wrote was *The Medicine Men* - an exposé of the drug industry. It made me very unpopular with the medical profession but sold quite well. I remember the paperback being piled up at railway stations. A series of novels I did for Macmillan under a pen name sold well and Pan did them in paperback. Three of my books got into the *Sunday Times* bestselling top ten. And quite a lot of foreign rights were sold. The first books I self-published were *Alice's Diary* and *The Village Cricket Tour* - both fiction. Both are still in print. *The Village Cricket Tour* has sold over 30,000 in hardback which isn't bad for a novel about cricket. One of my early novels, a book called *Mrs Caldicot's Cabbage War*, was made into a movie starring Pauline Collins.

Question 3.

There seems to be a continuous thread running through your books - cynicism towards the current established view on any subject you tackle - do you think this is a fair comment and did it originate with your views on medicine?

Answer

Yes, it's a fair comment. When I first started researching my early medical books I was shocked to discover just how much the establishment lies. My second discovery was that telling the truth isn't very popular. Over the years I've predicted just about every major development in medicine - and frequently warned about unreported hazards. Naturally, this hasn't made me popular with drug companies, doctors or politicians. I've been banned by just about every media outlet and these days it's extremely rare for any of my books to be reviewed anywhere - or for me to be interviewed. Journalists who claim to be open-minded tend to shy away from anyone who asks embarrassing questions or reveals embarrassing truths. The news most people watch on TV or read in their newspaper is Bowdlerised and sanitised; it doesn't bear much resemblance to the truth.

Question 4.

In 2002 you published *England Our England*. This was a fairly dramatic change in subject matter. Was there one reason for this or was it a steady build-up of dissatisfaction with the direction in which the country was heading?

Answer

I first got interested in the EU because of my researches into the world of medicine. I gradually realised that every trail I started to follow ended up in Brussels. And so campaigning against medical abuses had to involve the European Union. That led me to writing *England Our England*. I discovered that the EU planned to get rid of England completely. Hence the book. Most people have absolutely no idea what is going on in this country. Since then my interest in the wider aspects of geopolitics has exploded. I've written two books about the USA and a number of books about British politics.

Question 5.

Do you still enjoy writing and which of your books gave you most pleasure to write?

Answer

Yes, I do still enjoy writing. If I didn't I wouldn't do it. I couldn't possibly pick out one book as being `special'. It is often said that writers regard their books as children and in my case it's true. If you put something of yourself into a book then it's bound to be special. If you don't put something of yourself into a book then it will be insipid and bloodless rubbish.

Question 5.

You are a couple of years older than the NHS. Who is in better shape, you or the NHS?

Answer

The NHS is moribund. It is, to use that hideous, modern phrase which administrators use to restrict making financial payments to patients who are only terminally ill, `terminally, terminal'. The NHS is being killed by stupidity, incompetence and a complete and utter failure to understand the basic principles of healthcare. It's easy to blame drug companies, politicians and administrators (and I have frequently done so) but doctors are the main culprits. The NHS has been kept alive, though in an irreversible coma, for many years. The sooner it is put out of its misery the better for us all.

Question 6.

You hold some controversial views on amongst other things, doctors, nurses, hospitals, pharmaceutical companies, administrators, vaccinations, screening and radiotherapy. Do you have much support for your views in the medical establishment? Do you find many people agree but are afraid to speak out?

Answer

You may be surprised but the majority of doctors agree with me. My views are based on the available evidence - and common sense. Most doctors are nervous about supporting me in public. (Probably because they will lose their jobs if they do). But most agree with almost everything I write. I can substantiate every claim I've ever made. (And no one from the establishment who disagrees with me will dare debate with me in public.)

Question 7.

You express highly controversial anti-establishment views which are unpalatable to some yet self-evident to others. Why do you think you aren't held in high esteem?

Answer

Several reasons. First, I've made far too many enemies. Second, I've been too outspoken and honest. Third, the media in Britain is controlled by the establishment and very reluctant to publish material which asks significant questions. Fourth, I'm utterly useless at networking or promoting myself. The result of all this is that my books are pretty much ignored by the establishment in the UK but they are keenly welcomed abroad and published in over 20 languages. For example, *How To Stop Your Doctor Killing You* was a hit in China and I've just signed a contract for a Spanish edition of *Coleman's Laws* to be published for Spanish speaking Americans. None of that is `whingeing' by the way. I can and do whinge but that isn't it.

Question 8.

How do you avoid litigation?

Answer

By sticking to the truth.

Question 9.

Do you think that if you expressed your views in a less sensationalist manner - I am thinking now of the `are you eating cancer' advertisement - you would be taken more seriously?

Answer

No. My first book (*The Medicine Men*) was taken very seriously by the establishment. It got a full page in *The Guardian* and reviews in most of the other papers - plus 20 minutes on BBC1. My second book (*Paper Doctors*) also had a great critical response. (Though neither book sold many copies). But it became clear that I was exposing too many truths. My next serious books (*The Health Scandal* and *Betrayal of Trust*) were totally ignored. It was only then - after my books were gagged - that I became a little more adventurous in the way that I promoted my books. The `Are you eating cancer?' advert is based on a simple truth. The meat on your plate could well contain a lump of cancer if the animal from which the meat was taken was ill. The question may be unpalatable but it's worth asking. Another advertisement drawing attention to the fact that meat causes cancer (I have a mass of scientific evidence to prove this, of course) was banned by just about everyone - including *Private Eye*. The bottom line is that if I expressed my views in a more academic way I'd still be gagged - and I wouldn't sell any books either. One out of two ain't bad.

Question 10.

Do you consider yourself to be a campaigner?

Answer

I'm just a writer. I see myself primarily as a purveyor of truth - though a lot of my non-fiction books have a campaigning tone.

Question 11.

Why did you at some point discontinue treating patients and concentrate on writing?

Answer

In the early 1980s I had a great deal of trouble with the British Government's National Health Service. I refused to divulge my patients' diagnoses to bureaucrats - arguing that this information was confidential. I was disciplined and fined and warned that I would continue to be fined if I continued to put confidentiality above the requirements of the bureaucrats. I resigned from the health service and hung up my stethoscope. I felt that I could do more to `change the world' by writing than by struggling to practise in such an unsympathetic environment.

Question 12.

What is your opinion on the basic measures that a man must take in order to improve and maintain a good health?

Answer

I have gradually come to believe that diet is one of the most significant factors in the development of disease. But this again is a battle. Advertisements for my book *Food for Thought* were banned in the UK because I dared to tell people about the links between food and cancer. Dealing with stress is another vital factor - particularly since stress has such a powerful influence on the immune system. I was writing about stress in the mid 1970s - and was widely condemned by the medical establishment for daring to suggest that diseases such as high blood pressure might be related to stress.

Postscript 3: The Author

Vernon Coleman qualified as a doctor in 1970 and has worked both in hospitals and as a GP. He is still registered and licensed to practise as a GP principal. He has founded and organised many campaigns concerning iatrogenesis, drug addiction and the abuse of animals and has given evidence to committees at the House of Commons and House of Lords. Dr Coleman's campaigns have often proved successful. For example, after a 15 year campaign (which started in 1973) he eventually persuaded the British Government to introduce stricter controls governing the prescribing of benzodiazepine tranquillisers. `Dr Vernon Coleman's articles, to which I refer with approval, raised concern about these important matters,' said the Parliamentary Secretary for Health in the House of Commons in 1988.

He has worked as a columnist for numerous national newspapers including *The Sun*, *The Daily Star*, *The Sunday Express* and *The People* and has written columns for over 50 regional newspapers. His columns and articles have appeared in newspapers and magazines around the world. He has contributed articles to hundreds of other publications including *The Sunday Times, Observer, Guardian, Daily Telegraph, Sunday Telegraph, Daily Express, Daily Mail, Mail on Sunday, Daily Mirror, Sunday Mirror, Punch, Woman, Woman's Own, The Lady, Spectator* and *British Medical Journal*. He was the founding editor of the *British Clinical Journal*. He was for some years one of the highest paid columnists in Britain.

He has presented numerous programmes on television and radio and was the original breakfast television doctor. He was television's first agony uncle (on BBC1's The Afternoon Show). He has presented three TV series based on his bestselling book *Bodypower*. In the now long-gone days when producers and editors were less wary of annoying the establishment he was a regular broadcaster on radio and television.

His books have been published in the UK by *Arrow, Pan, Penguin, Corgi, Mandarin, Star, Piatkus, RKP, Thames* and *Hudson, Sidgwick and Jackson, Macmillan* and many other leading publishing houses. His books have been translated into 25 languages, and English versions sell in America, Australia, Canada and South Africa as well as the UK. Several have appeared on both the *Sunday Times* and *Bookseller* bestseller lists. He has written over 100 books which have, together, sold over two million copies in the UK alone. His novel *Mrs Caldicot's Cabbage War* has been filmed and is, like many of his other novels, available in an audio version. He has co-written four books with his wife, Donna Antoinette Coleman.

He has never had a proper job (in the sense of working for someone else in regular, paid employment, with a cheque or pay packet at the end of the week or month) but he has had freelance and temporary employment in many forms. He has, for example, had paid employment as: magician's assistant, postman, fish delivery van driver, production line worker, chemical laboratory assistant, author, publisher, draughtsman, meals on wheels driver, feature writer, drama critic, book reviewer, columnist, surgeon, police surgeon, industrial medical officer, social worker, nightclub operator, property developer, magazine editor, general practitioner, private doctor, television presenter, radio presenter, agony aunt, university lecturer, casualty doctor and care home assistant. Much to his (and probably also to their) surprise, he has given evidence to committees in the House of Commons and the House of Lords. Whether they took any notice of what he had to say is doubtful. They did not fall asleep.

Today, he likes books, films, cafés and writing. He writes, reads and collects books and has a larger library than most towns. A list of his favourite authors would require another book. He has never been much of an athlete, though he once won a certificate for swimming a width of the public baths in Walsall (which was, at the time, in Staffordshire but has now, apparently, been moved elsewhere).

He doesn't like yappy dogs, big snarly dogs with saliva dripping from their fangs or people who think that wearing a uniform automatically gives them status and rights over everyone else. He likes trains, dislikes planes and used to like cars until idiots invented speed cameras, bus lanes and car parks where the spaces are so narrow that only the slimmest of vehicles will fit in.

He is inordinately fond of cats, likes pens and notebooks and used to enjoy watching cricket until the authorities sold out and allowed people to paint slogans on the grass. His interests include animals, photography, drawing, chess, backgammon, cinema, philately, billiards, sitting in cafés and on benches and collecting Napoleana and old books that were written and published before dustwrappers were invented. He likes log fires and bonfires, motor racing and music by Beethoven, Mozart and Mahler and dislikes politicians, bureaucrats and cauliflower cheese. He likes videos but loathes DVDs. His favourite 12 people in history include (in no particular order): Daniel Defoe, Che Guevera, Napoleon Bonaparte, W. G. Grace, William Cobbett, Thomas Paine, John Lilburne, Aphra Behn, P. G. Wodehouse, Jerome K. Jerome, Francis Drake and Walter Ralegh all of whom had more than it takes and most of whom were English. What an unbeatable team they would have made. Grace and Bonaparte opening the batting and Drake and Ralegh opening the bowling. Gilles Villeneuve would bring on the drinks, though would probably spill more than he delivered.

Vernon Coleman lives in the delightful if isolated village of Bilbury in Devon and enjoys malt whisky, toasted muffins and old films. He is devoted to Donna Antoinette, the Welsh Princess, who is the kindest, sweetest, most sensitive woman a man could hope to meet and who, as an undeserved but welcome bonus, makes the very best roast parsnips on the planet. He says that gourmands and gourmets would come from far and wide if they knew what they were missing but admits that since he and his pal Thumper Robinson took down the road signs (in order to discourage tourists travelling to Bilbury on coaches) the village where he lives has become exceedingly difficult to find.

Note:

For a full list of books by Vernon Coleman please visit http://www.vernoncoleman.com/ or Amazon Author Central. d

Printed in Great Britain
by Amazon